INNOVATIONS IN
NURSING EDUCATION
ADMINISTRATION

Innovations

in

Nursing Education Administration √

A Tribute to Dean Billye J. Brown, EdD

Edited by

Mabel A. Wandelt, PhD, FAAN
Professor Emeritus
University of Texas at Austin

Betty J. Thomas, MNSc, RN, CNAA
Director, Tuft and Associates
Chicago, Illinois

Pub. No. 15-2344

 National League for Nursing · New York

Copyright © 1990 by
National League for Nursing
350 Hudson Street
New York, NY 10014

The views expressed in this book reflect those
of the authors and do not necessarily reflect the
official views of the National League for
Nursing.

ISBN 0-88737-492-1

Manufactured in the United States of America

Innovation: Everyone is in favor of it as long as it is not accompanied by change.

Sy Axelrod
University of Michigan
School of Public Health
Findings (Winter 1987–88)

DEDICATION

This work is dedicated to Billye J. Brown, EdD, RN, FAAN, on the occasion of her retirement as founding dean of the University of Texas at Austin School of Nursing. It is meant to serve as a reminder of Dean Brown's constant and continuing interest in the field of nursing education and educational administration.

CONTENTS

XI. ALUMNI AND PUBLIC RELATIONS

XII. DREAMS

APPENDIX A

CONTRIBUTORS' AFFILIATION

Balcerski, Judith A., PhD, RN, Dean and Professor [30]*
    School of Nursing
    Barry University
    Miami Shores, FL

Barnum, Barbara J., PhD, RN, FAAN, Editor, *Nursing & Health Care*,
    National League for Nursing
    New York, NY [14, 22, 32]

Carty, Rita M., DNSc, RN, FAAN, Dean [50]
    School of Nursing
    George Mason University
    Fairfax, VA

Castiglia, Patricia T., PhD, RN, Dean [39]
    College of Nursing and Allied Health
    University of Texas
    El Paso, TX

Chamings, Patricia A., PhD, RN, CNA, Dean and Professor [34]
    School of Nursing
    University of North Carolina at Greensboro
    Greensboro, NC

Chickadonz, Grace H., PhD, RN, Dean and Professor [41]
    College of Nursing
    Syracuse University
    Syracuse, NY

---

* Indicates contribution chapter number(s).

Christman, Luther, PhD, RN, FAAN, Dean Emeritus [52, 63]
    College of Nursing
    Rush University
    Chicago, IL

Clemence, Barbara A., DNSc, RN, President and Dean [47]
    Research College of Nursing
    Kansas City, MO

Conway, Mary E., PhD, FAAN, Dean [38]
    School of Nursing
    Medical College of Georgia
    Augusta, GA

Conway-Welch, Colleen, PhD, CNM, FAAN, Dean and Professor [35]
    School of Nursing
    Vanderbilt University
    Nashville, TN

Diers, Donna, MSN, RN, FAAN, Professor [33]
    School of Nursing
    Yale University
    New Haven, CT

Drennan, Phyllis, PhD, Dean and Professor [43]
    School of Nursing
    University of Missouri
    Columbia, MO

Edwards, Doris S., EdD, RN, Dean and Professor [16]
    School of Nursing
    Capital University
    Columbus, OH

Feldman, Harriet R., PhD, RN, Chairperson [26]
    Department of Nursing
    Fairleigh Dickinson University
    Rutherford, NJ

Felton, Geraldene, EdD, RN, FAAN, Professor and Dean [37, 60]
    College of Nursing
    University of Iowa
    Iowa City, IA

Fitzpatrick, M. Louise, EdD, RN, FAAN, Dean and Professor [6]
    College of Nursing
    Villanova University
    Villanova, PA

Ford, Loretta C., EdD, RN, FAAN, Professor; Dean and Director
        of Nursing [53, 64]
    University of Rochester Medical Center
    Rochester, NY

Goldberg, Enid, PhD, RN, Dean and Professor [48, 55]
School of Nursing
University of Pittsburgh
Pittsburgh, PA

Goodman, Lillian R., EdD, RN, Chairperson/Professor [24]
Department of Nursing
Worcester State College
Worcester, MA

Gray, Carol J., EdD, RN, Dean [44]
School of Nursing
Johns Hopkins University
Baltimore, MD

Gudmundsen, Anne, PhD, RN, Professor of Nursing
and Former Dean [20]
College of Nursing
Texas Woman's University
Denton, TX

Haus, Barbara F., EdD, RN, Chairperson [49]
Department of Nursing
Albright College
Reading, PA

Hawken, Patty, PhD, RN, Dean and Professor [19]
School of Nursing
Health Science Center at San Antonio
University of Texas
San Antonio, TX

Hechenberger, Nan B., PhD, Dean and Professor [42]
School of Nursing
University of Maryland
Baltimore, MD

Hegyvary, Sue T., PhD, FAAN, Professor and Dean [29]
School of Nursing
University of Washington
Seattle, WA

Henderson, Frances C., EdD, RN, Director [8]
Division of Nursing
Alcorn State University
Natchez, MS

Hill, Betty J., PhD, RN, Dean [7]
School of Nursing and Allied Health Sciences
Northern Michigan University
Marquette, MI

Hoff, Julienne, PhD, RN, Dean [10]
Division of Nursing and Health
Madonna College
Livonia, MI

Hott, Jacqueline Rose, CS, PhD, RN, FAAN, Dean and Professor [12, 61]
Marion A. Buckley School of Nursing
Adelphi University
Garden City, NY

Krafft, Sandra, EdD, RN, Chairperson [5]
Department of Health Sciences
Wilmington College
New Castle, DE

Lancaster, Jeanette, PhD, RN, FAAN, Dean and Professor [23]
School of Nursing
Wright State University
Dayton, OH

Lang, Norma M., PhD, RN, FAAN, Dean and Professor [28]
School of Nursing
University of Wisconsin
Milwaukee, WI

Lange, Crystal M., PhD, RN, FAAN, Dean and Professor [27]
College of Nursing
Saginaw Valley State University
University Center, MI

Leifson, June, PhD, MS, RN, Dean and Professor [46]
College of Nursing
Brigham Young University
Provo, UT

Murillo-Rohde, Ildaura, PhD, RN, CS, FAAN, Dean and Professor
Emeritus [31, 62]
College of Nursing
State University of New York
Brooklyn, NY

Mutzebaugh, Carole A., EdD, RN, Former Chair [11]
Department of Nursing
University of Southern Colorado
Pueblo, CO

O'Koren, Marie L., EdD, Dean Emerita [45]
School of Nursing
University of Alabama
Birmingham, AL

Opitz, Margaret (Peggy) G., EdD, RN, Head [25]
Department of Nursing
North Georgia College
Dahlonega, GA

Ostmoe, Patricia M., PhD, RN, Dean [3]
School of Nursing
University of Wisconsin
Eau Claire, WI

Pickard, Myrna R., EdD, RN, Dean and Professor of Nursing [4]
School of Nursing
University of Texas
Arlington, TX

Rand, Joella M., PhD, RN, Dean [1]
College of Nursing
Alfred University
Alfred, NY

Roehm, Maryanne E., EdD, RN, Professor and Dean [58]
School of Nursing
Indiana University
Terre Haute, IN

Sands, Rosetta F., PhD, RN, Dean [17]
School of Health Professions and Nursing
William Paterson College of New Jersey
Wayne, NJ

Saucier, Karen A., PhD, RN, Dean [9, 21]
School of Nursing
Delta State University
Cleveland, MS

Schaefer, Marguerite J., DSc [56]
Health Education and Management Consultant
Pittsburgh, PA

Schlotfeldt, Rozella M., PhD, FAAN, Dean Emeritus [57]
Frances Payne Bolton School of Nursing
Case-Western Reserve University
Cleveland, OH

Shannon, Anna M., DNS, RN, FAAN, Dean [2]
College of Nursing
Montana State University
Bozeman, MT

Shetland, Margaret L., PhD, RN, Dean and Professor Emeritus [36]
College of Nursing
Wayne State University
Detroit, MI

Smith, Dorothy M., RN, Dean Emeritus [51]
    College of Nursing
    Chief of Nursing Staff, Shands Hospital
    University of Florida
    Gainesville, FL

Sorensen, Gladys, EdD, RN, FAAN, Dean Emerita and Professor
        Emerita [54]
    College of Nursing
    University of Arizona
    Tucson, AZ

Speer, Justine J., PhD, RN, Dean [59]
    School of Nursing
    University of Louisville
    Louisville, KY

Stecchi, Janice M., EdD, RN, Professor and Chairperson [13]
    Department of Nursing
    University of Lowell
    Lowell, MA

Styles, Margretta M., EdD, RN, FAAN, Livingston Professor of Nursing
        [15]
    School of Nursing
    University of California
    San Francisco, CA

Watson, Jean, PhD, RN, FAAN, Dean and Professor, Associate
        Director [18]
    Department of Nursing, University Hospital
    Director, Center of Human Caring
    University of Colorado Health Sciences Center
    Denver, CO

Yeaworth, Rosalee C., PhD, RN, Dean and Professor of Nursing [40]
    College of Nursing
    University of Nebraska Medical Center
    Omaha, NE

CONTRIBUTORS' COMMENTS: A MULTIPLE DEDICATION

I applaud your creative approach in honoring Dr. Billye J. Brown. She is a most well-loved and respected nursing leader. The book should be well received as well as a treasure for all nurses. I look forward to its publication debut.

I am pleased to submit the attached description of one of the simplest, yet one of the most effective things I have done as dean. I look forward to reading the best ideas of my colleagues throughout the nation.

Thank you for asking me to contribute to a book which is dedicated to Dean Billye J. Brown. I believe your idea of a compendium of information about the business of administration in honor of Dean Brown is inspired.

My entry is not exactly an innovation, but it is a concept that has been extremely valuable to the viability of our school of nursing.

What a marvelous idea that will recognize Dr. Brown's career in nursing. I am pleased to submit an "idea" and look forward to reading the innovations of other administrators.

As a new Dean (I feel that way, although it is going on three years since I was appointed), I appreciate the challenge you gave me when you asked me to reminisce and to write a brief description of the best innovation I have implemented as dean. This may not be the best, but it has been the most challenging and most time-consuming.

I am pleased to be asked to share in this endeavor. I am enclosing my very best innovation. It was remarkably successful in instituting our research thrust and in giving our college a focus—rural nursing. I'll look forward to seeing the compilation of innovations. The idea is a splendid one for recognizing Dean Brown's many contributions.

What a wonderful way to honor Dr. Brown! I am enclosing my contribution to the collection and have also added a list of suggestions which might be of assistance to a new dean.

Here are my "Reminiscence" and "My Dream." They may not be much, but I think they will do. I think the project you are doing is a great one, not only for Billye but also for the profession as a whole.

I hope that the enclosed narrative adds something to what I am sure will be a delightful and useful collection of administrative insights.

April 1989

PREFACE

This compendium, made up of contributions from more than fifty administrators of schools of nursing, is meant to interest and help several groups of nurses. It is foremost directed to students of nursing educational administration who should find it a valuable reference.

Since experience is an excellent teacher, the innovations, ideas, and dreams of those who implemented or wanted to implement the described events may serve as examples or catalysts for future nursing deans as well as those who currently hold that position.

The descriptions of administrative actions are divided into such categories as curriculum, faculty support, uniting practice and education, alumni, public relations, and community collaboration. In all the designated categories, Dean Brown has been an exemplary leader and outstanding role model for the profession.

Not only did she lead the University of Texas at Austin School of Nursing to become one of the most widely recognized and prestigious schools in the United States, but she also served the nursing profession as president or top executive volunteer in such organizations as the American Nurses' Association, the American Association of Colleges of Nursing, Sigma Theta Tau International, the National League for Nursing, and the American Academy of Nursing.

Although recognized for her excellent abilities as a fund raiser, Dr. Brown has always valued most her opportunity to influence student nurses at all stages of their educational processes. In that spirit of influential sharing, this book has been developed and dedicated in her honor.

We are deeply grateful to the contributing nursing deans who, like Dean Brown, have shared their own knowledge, experience, and wisdom.

Mabel A. Wandelt
Betty J. Thomas

Part I

OUTREACH PROGRAMS

1

ATTENTION TO HUMAN AND TECHNICAL FACTORS

Joella M. Rand

Although outreach programming and distance learning have been a part of the corporate environment for decades, it is one of the major innovations at Alfred University College of Nursing. The nursing college is the first college within the university to initiate such an activity. The program started in response to a need to reach learners who could not travel to the traditional classroom setting and to provide a mechanism to link educationally the main campus of Alfred University, located in a rural setting, with a nursing division located in a metropolitan area. There is also a need to create a mechanism whereby full-time, expert faculty could interact with all populations the College of Nursing serves: traditional nursing students, students pursuing a second career in nursing, and RN students.

The response to the need has been developed in the context of the College of Nursing's emphasis on excellence, opportunity, accountability, and adaptability. The initial effort was to offer courses through audio conferencing with preproduced video with a future plan to develop computer conferencing and communication satellite learning opportunities.

Teleconferencing offers the capacity for group discussion oriented toward application of information from different areas and subsequent conversion to knowledge. Students from different geographic locations bring depth and breadth of enthusiasm and perspective to the group learning process. The technique fosters the discovery of knowledge in a group setting. Successful implementation is the result of careful and

3

continual attention to both the human factor and the technical factor sides of the operation. To date, student response has been very positive, with students requesting to have an opportunity to participate in the experience.

On the human factor side, teaching strategies have been adapted with all students receiving the same materials. Packets of materials for participants and preproduced video are prepared and on-site in advance of the class meeting. There is an effort to include all students in the discussion, with a definite bias toward interaction. Classes are kept small to facilitate interaction and personal opportunity and accountability. A picture of each student is available in each site. Faculty development and networking among college departments, particularly the Communications Department, is encouraged.

From the technical side, an evaluation system for students is in place to provide continual feedback. Arrangements for technical equipment are in place prior to each session and each student is oriented to the use of equipment with appropriate etiquette for on-line conversation. Students are further supported with personal telephone contacts and use of off-line activities and materials prepared and received in advance. Two-way audio feedback gives immediacy to fostering support of the distance learner.

Nursing has taken the lead in distance learning in our university and it is a proud achievement. While the project is still developing and will continue to be refined both in the technical and human factor realities, the hope is that with nursing in the lead position, other departments will join in utilizing the latest communication technology and put in place a full-scale satellite communication system for distance learning at Alfred University.

2

GRADUATE EDUCATION AND FACULTY RESEARCH: TWO FOR THE PRICE OF ONE

Anna M. Shannon

At a time when resources were few, faculty research was minimal, and an opportunity arose for modifying the graduate program, the Two for One program was conceived and implemented. The changed graduate program focused on the needs of the state (rural) and, since there was no research literature about rural nursing, the program's focus was on identifying the health care needs in sparsely populated areas. Through prescriptive student course assignments using an ethnographic approach to data collection, information was systematically gathered about perceptions of health and health care needs in rural towns. These data then constituted a pool for content analysis by a faculty group to begin generation of a rural nursing theory and development of hypotheses for further research.

The graduate students learned a systematic approach (ethnographic inquiry) to assess health care needs and the faculty group gained a store of qualitative data about health and health care delivery. Since the graduate program was rotated among the extended campuses of the college, data now exist from towns all over the state, representing different subcultures, occupations, age groups, and levels of population density. The faculty group interested in this project gained a data set, collegial support from a common interest, and development of research skills. Faculty research has increased markedly.

The next phase of this project will use the same methodology, except key concepts derived from the first efforts that are probably relevant to rural nursing will be selected (i.e., isolation). These concepts will then form the basis of the student course assignments whereby, through ethnographic interviews, the salient factors to rural nursing will be assessed. Thus will begin the process of concept validation. Again, the students will benefit by learning a systematic approach for assessing health care needs and the faculty group will gain further refinement of the data set.

3

A PROGRAM'S NUMBER AND VARIETY OF ELEMENTS

Patricia M. Ostmoe

The University of Wisconsin–Eau Claire School of Nursing, under the leadership of the dean, embarked in 1986 on one of its most challenging innovations to date. In an effort to prepare more baccalaureate degreed nurses for the rural areas of central Wisconsin and to accommodate the educational needs of geographically bound, non-traditional students, we established a basic baccalaureate nursing program at an off-campus site located 85 miles from the main campus. The program is offered in cooperation with two 2-year campuses, another 4-year institution, and a hospital that previously administered a 3-year diploma school of nursing.

The model that guided the development of the program incorporated aspects of three traditional outreach program models previously documented in the literature. These include the satellite model, the cooperative model, and the interinstitutional model. The design of this "multi-model" outreach nursing program included the following components: a separate-but-equal-in-quality curriculum offered at the off-campus site, faculty hired for the off-campus site after completion of a year-long on-campus orientation, on-campus faculty travel to the off-campus site for instructional purposes, use of audiographic telecommunications teaching strategies, off-campus faculty travel to the main campus for participation in university governance, recruitment and advisement of students by all participating educational institutions, partial funding support for the program by the hospital, provision of non-nursing course by the 4-year and

2-year campuses, availability of instructional facilities at the cooperating institutions, sharing of financial aid administration, and provision of student scholarship support through the hospital.

The program demonstrates unprecedented cooperation between four separate educational institutions and a private nonprofit health care agency. Its establishment facilitated the closing of a diploma school of nursing without disrupting the supply of registered nurses to a rural area and, serendipitously, the initiation of the program offset unanticipated declines in on-campus enrollments.

4

CONTINUING EDUCATION FOR RURAL HEALTH CARE

Myrna R. Pickard

The best innovation that I have implemented as a dean has been our rural outreach program. This program was initiated in 1975 with the assistance of a grant from the Sid Richardson Foundation. The original purpose was to provide continuing education programs for 26 small hospitals within a 2-hour driving range of Fort Worth, Texas. We received funding of $150,000 for 3 years and we developed good working relationships with our rural colleagues in health care. When the Sid Richardson grant ended in 1978, we were able to get line item state funding for the project and it has continued to the present time. The major goal continues to be continuing education offerings to the small rural hospitals, but we have expanded the program in a number of ways. We conduct some regional programs in addition to the on-site continuing education programs and we have included long-term care, home care, and other health care personnel.

Another expansion of the program resulted in involving graduate students in the provision of services including consultation. Several of the graduate faculty agreed to have the rural continuing education or consulting projects as an option for a course assignment. The result was most rewarding. The majority of the graduate students had never been involved in rural health care and they were amazed at the difference between urban and rural. They found it rewarding and frustrating. They were unable to make definite plans because, with a very small staff, changes have to be made at the last minute. They also found that the receptivity was extremely positive: one graduate student who did a consultation project was actually hired by the rural hospital.

Our future plans involve the offering of a rural nursing elective for undergraduate students. We have commitments from several rural agencies to provide room and board for the students to spend an intense period of time in their community. Nursing personnel view this experience as a recruitment opportunity.

We believe this is one small way to assist with the rural health care crisis and it has been a rewarding experience.

5

FACULTY UTILIZATION AT A SATELLITE SITE

Sandra Krafft

Several years ago a decision was made by our small liberal arts college to respond to a frequently expressed community need—that of offering reasonable access to baccalaureate education to registered nurses.

A feasibility study was conducted that not only identified a substantial population desiring this education but also targeted two geographic clusters of potential students approximately 100 miles apart. One cluster was located in the vicinity of our main campus near a mid-size city in the most populated area of the state and the other was in a rural area in the southern portion of the state. The college already offered other programs at the satellite location in this area.

The objective of implementing a new program at two sites with minimal staffing certainly caused many sleepless nights, but it was well worth the effort $3\frac{1}{2}$ years later when we could announce to our very first graduating class that they had graduated from a fully accredited baccalaureate nursing program.

I believe in retrospect that several important administrative decisions were fundamental to the program's success. The first of these was a year devoted to curriculum planning, policy development, and implementation methodology. This was accomplished by the chairperson and one full-time faculty member prior to the admission of students into the nursing component.

Second, a decision to base the second full-time faculty member at the rural site rather than the main campus proved to be extremely beneficial.

11

This provided a general "presence" in the community and greatly facilitated student advisement and administration of testing, etc.

Third, faculty were hired to reflect not only a variety of clinical specialties but also areas of additional expertise, i.e., program evaluation, outcomes assessment, and curriculum development.

Fourth, these four faculty were absolutely committed to providing comparable services and exposure to a variety of faculty at both locations rather than the assignment of one or two individuals to each site.

During the early planning and implementation phases, the department members were also intensely involved in the accreditation process. The ambitious goals demanded much of the four individuals involved. Therefore, my goal was to facilitate the development of a creative faculty utilization plan that would allow the department to offer comparable programs at each site and to minimize faculty burn-out. Key elements in this plan included gaining administrative approval for considering travel time (4 hours round trip) as 4 contact hours equal to classroom or clinical teaching time. Travel expenses were reimbursed and overnight lodging provided if necessary. Theory courses were more conducive for long-distance travel but in a few instances arrangements were also made for clinical courses. Travel was initially limited to a maximum of two courses per year, with the development of a long-range plan to decrease this to once per year. (This will be realized this fall following the graduation of the second class.)

As many department meetings as possible were held at a location midway between the two sites to equalize travel among all faculty. Last but not least, participatory development of the teaching schedule at each site allowed consideration of the needs and preferences of each faculty member.

In summary, travel is possible, travel is time, travel is difficult, and travel must be fairly compensated in order for travel to work.

Part II

NATURE OF NURSING FOR OTHER PROFESSIONS

6

COLLEAGUES IN OTHER PROFESSIONS EXPERIENCE EDUCATION IN NURSING

M. Louise Fitzpatrick

The most important innovation that I have instituted since becoming a dean, 11 years ago, is to deliberately plan the education of key administrators and others within the university community of nursing.

We are a private, church-related, comprehensive university of approximately 10,000 students, of which 6,500 are undergraduates. Professional schools within our institution include Colleges of Engineering, Law, and Business. Nursing is the only health profession for which we prepare our students.

Although our College of Nursing was celebrating its twenty-fifth anniversary when I became dean in 1978, it soon became apparent that the perception of nursing and nursing education by administrators and faculty from other disciplines was "fixed" at about 1960. The developments in health care, the financial concerns that surround it, and the burgeoning technology that affect it were intellectually accepted by my academic colleagues. Yet, I realized that creating new opportunities for informing them about nursing, nursing education, and the changing health care scene would be critical if we were to be well positioned for the development and maturation of our college.

In some respects, the educational process that has evolved occurred quite naturally. In other respects, it was designed. The important point is that it has all been planned. From the outset, my objective was clear. The College of Nursing, its administration, faculty, and students needed to create opportunities to help others interpret the goals of the profession

15

and in particular the goals and agenda of our college. Only in this way could we create an interest in and a lasting support for our work.

Examples of what we have done are not necessarily unique, but the systematic strategy employed is, I believe, innovative. Being a public health nurse at heart, I now recognize that these efforts have really been based on the preventive approach and they have built up our immunity against difficulty with our administration and trustees. Despite lower enrollments, the need to expend more resources to recruit students, the need to replace retirees with more qualified faculty who must be paid higher salaries, and the need to maintain low student/faculty clinical ratios which make nursing education expensive, we have been better understood and supported because we took the initiative to educate and inform those who hold the power to influence our future as a College of Nursing.

We are fortunate that our university's mission and philosophy support nursing as integral to institutional goals. But in today's world, that alone is not enough. Having an increasingly well informed central administration and university community has helped to develop a better understanding of the challenges we face and the needs we have as a college, and this has increased support for what we do to develop even further.

What is this educational strategy? Actually, it has been a simple plan, though varied in approach and effective for the college. Top-level administrators at the time of their appointment have been invited to meet with us to learn about our program and have then been given the opportunity to visit clinical facilities with us when our faculty and students are engaged in the clinical teaching-learning process. This experience has incalculable value in helping non-nurses understand what students and faculty do in the clinical laboratory, what the health care environment is like, and what variables drive our educational programs. Because most faculty from other disciplines would not be in a position to visit the clinical settings with us, we host a reception and preview the media presentations that are used for student recruitment, etc., as well as other appropriate materials that can inform people about the field. Our top-level administrators, including the president, have also visited the clinical setting.

Another effective approach has been a deliberate plan to provide *pro bono* services for the campus community. From our annual Health Fair, to teaching CPR to the Security Department, to providing services on health related topics for the Student Life Department, College of Nursing faculty and students have seized some opportunities and created others to demonstrate what nurses do beyond their traditional roles. Health consultation and referrals are frequently part of what we provide to those who seek our advice.

Our faculty use their opportunities on university-wide committees to clarify and describe what the educational process in nursing entails and the reasons for it. Whenever possible, we attempt to draw parallels between what we do and those things which are familiar to people in other disciplines. In these ways, we find the "common ground." Consequences of this, long term, can also lead to possibilities for collaborative efforts in academic programs and in the scholarly work of faculty and students.

The College of Nursing's standing committees make a deliberate effort to communicate with parallel committees within the structure of the university senate or with university offices that are important to us in interpreting our college to the public. One such relationship exists between our college's public relations committee and the university's Office of University Relations and Public Information.

If nursing is supported and understood on our campus, it is because we make a concerted effort to inform and educate our colleagues. We do not just hope that it will naturally happen. When you are the only health profession and clinical practice field on a campus, this kind of endeavor can make the difference between heath and illness for a college of nursing.

I am not sure if what we have done is innovative. But it has been part of my plan for the college and it has certainly been effective.

7

ORIENTING A NEW ACADEMIC VP

Betty J. Hill

The process of orienting or socializing a new academic vice president regarding the discipline of nursing, particularly an academic VP who was formerly a dean of arts and science, as so many are, is a challenging task for a nursing dean. One of the ways I have attempted to do this in addition to making regular informational appointments with a new academic VP is to have the VP don a laboratory jacket and spend a full day with me in an acute-care hospital where our senior nursing students are doing their management clinical experience.

The planned visit to an acute-care hospital to observe senior student nurses in practice and nursing faculty teaching in that setting brings to focus in a dramatic way the facts that:

1. Nursing is one of the few disciplines in a university that attempts to prepare new graduates to function in real, high-risk, high-tech, human care environments and to assume serious responsibilities for human life in 4 or less years of education post high school.

2. Nursing faculty must be competent and current-with-technology practitioners to safely and effectively accomplish the first item on this list. In addition to clinical competence, nursing faculty must meet the other requirements of being university professors, such as teaching, service, and scholarship.

Invariably a new academic VP is impressed by the practice skills of our senior student nurses and by the very challenging teaching/learning environments in which nursing faculty must function. Such an experience helps a great deal when a nursing dean later discusses staffing with a new academic VP and the reasons for small student-teacher ratios, particularly in acute-care clinics.

This innoculation experience with a new academic VP may have to be repeated within 1 or 2 years, and probably the experience should be extended to other members of a university's central administration, including the president and members of the board of governors. This may help the university decision makers to realize why the nursing department is different from and more expensive than, say, the biology department.

Another important reason why the academic VP and others should observe an acute-care setting when nursing students are there is so university administrators might learn to value the technical level and the social importance of the work that nurses, including student nurses and new graduates, contribute to the health-care enterprise. I know such an experience continues to amaze and impress this nursing dean, and the clinical visit experience also reminds me of why I am proud to be a nursing education administrator.

Part III

LISTINGS

8

IF

Frances C. Henderson

If you can keep your focus when all about you are losing theirs and
blaming it on administration,

If you can chair all sorts of meetings and not lose an agenda,

If you can answer calls and follow-up on telephone messages
promptly,

If you can travel to city after city and still know where you are and
why,

If you can pass the test of faculty, staff, students, and your
superiors,

If you can sort your mail and respond to essential communiques
with speed,

If you can mark your calendar without one double booking,

If you can smile when budget time is near,

If you can kindle a spark of enthusiasm from those who doubt you,

If you can sleep four hours each night and not feel guilty for having
slept,

If you can but travel to meeting destinations on weekends and not
take a suitcase full of papers,

If you can serve on ten committees and not forget each charge,

If you can laugh at you and not take yourself for granted while others seem to do so with expertise,

If you can be assertive enough to win negotiations without the use of tactics bordering on aggression,

If you can actively listen to faculty, staff, and students and still remain objective,

If you can find quality time to spend with family and friends and not forget their birthdays,

If you can prepare for accreditation and yet serve on an accreditation team,

If you can but convince yourself at times that things are really not quite as bad as they seem,

If you can recruit faculty and students when the pool gets mighty slim,

If you can greet your graduates and call them each by name,

If you can make a difference in the community and manage to convince them that it really is their town,

If you can coordinate the construction of buildings instead of trying to leap over them in a single bound,

If you can read all professional nursing and nursing-related journals and still fancy reading a juicy novel every night,

If you can write for publication and enthusiastically encourage others to do the same,

If you can proof proposals, manuscripts, and reports and still have time for a friendly scrabble game,

If you can write a speech and remember every word that is in it,

If you can change your plans so as to attend to urgent priorities on the spur of just one minute,

If you can obtain external funding to transform dreams into realities without ever doubting that you can,

If you can mentor others and yet yourself be mentored with aplomb,

If you can argue a salient point and not be argumentative,

If you can risk and have no fear of risking,

If you can follow suit and not make the past your ruler,

If you can keep your cool when the president's call catches you by surprise yet find the words to respond with natural finesse,

If you can quote enrollment figures without batting an eye or letting on that it really is an educated guess,

If you can teach and learn, do and be, love and laugh, despair, rejoice, and see far into the future and still have time for fun,

If you can acknowledge differences in opinion without compromising your own beliefs in excellence,

If you can balance participatory management for the good of the organization with enough authority for credibility and not give up in your quest,

If you can use your power to empower others to always do their best,

Then you are a nursing administrator *par excellence*, standing head and shoulders along with all the rest.

9

TEN SUGGESTIONS FOR A
NEW DEAN IN A SMALL SCHOOL
OF NURSING

Karen A. Saucier

1. Learn to use your trash can; it can be an important filing mechanism.

2. Hire an exceptional secretary and delegate.

3. Learn to close your door without feeling guilty (this also applies to having your phone calls held).

4. Share administrative duties with your faculty, especially those interested in a career in administration (class scheduling, official university representation, proofreading of official materials, etc.).

5. Develop friendships *outside* of the School of Nursing; seek female administrative colleagues as mentors and consultants.

6. Keep your door open to all faculty and student problems, even when they seem relatively unimportant to you (use judgment as to seriousness of problem—see 3).

7. Learn to say no to projects you are *not* interested in although they might look good on your vita (you will have many projects to choose from which you are interested in—many more than you can imagine).

8. Attend at least one national nursing meeting a year, specifically for administrators, the collegial relationships will be very valuable in assisting you with problems and solutions (do this even if you have to pay for it yourself—the pay-off will be significant).

9. Develop relationships with the other deans in the university; learn from their perspectives and experiences in a non-nursing academic field.

10. Make time for yourself; avoid weekend work and find diversionary activities (this is the hardest rule to keep!).

Part IV

COMMUNICATIONS WITHIN THE SCHOOL OF NURSING

10

THE MONDAY MEMO: AN EFFECTIVE FACULTY AND STUDENT COMMUNICATION TOOL

Julienne Hoff

I was 3 months into a new deanship position, and despite warm faculty relations and an open-door policy, I felt that I was not communicating with the faculty on a regular, personal basis. Memos were one way of informing, reminding, and/or congratulating them, but excessive memos were costly, both in terms of time and resources. I decided to try something that had worked well in my previous position as dean: I initiated a weekly newsletter to faculty.

The Monday Memo is a simple, typed, and photocopied one- or two-page newsletter that I write each week to faculty. It contains most items of information that used to be put in individual memos and serves to remind faculty of meetings, ask for assistance or input with projects, and share times of personal or professional interest regarding faculty and staff. This last area is of particular importance to me. I can give recognition immediately to faculty publications or presentations, announce births of sons, daughters, or grandchildren, and ask for prayers when a personal illness or family death occurs. The *Memo* is printed on the some color paper each week, and it is in each faculty member's mailbox by 8:00 a.m. each Monday morning.

Faculty response has been extremely positive. They like the short, direct and regular communication system and know they can count on being kept up with the news each week. They also know that if they do not read the *Memo*, they might miss something because repetitive memos are not issued. Most important, though, faculty appreciate the feeling of communicating with me directly, and I feel that each week I have a chance to talk with them.

The real success of the *Memo* was apparent to me when the faculty suggested that I issue a student version of the *Memo* each week to facilitate the kind of communication and open relationship it had created for them. After a year of writing the student *Monday Memo*, I can say that it has been equally positive. Students seem to feel very much at ease with me, and are comfortable stopping in to talk if my door is open. Faculty and students often contribute notices and faculty no longer have to use the first 10 minutes of a class period making general announcements.

The Monday Memo has been one of the most effective innovations I have made. Sometimes it almost writes itself, because I have so many contributions; other times it is not so easy. Every Thursday or Friday I must find time to put the newsletters together, but the time is truly worth it. I am in touch with the two most important groups I serve, and they know they are in touch with me. I strongly recommend it as a simple, cost-effective method of moving beyond the dean's office on a regular basis.

11

CONVOCATION

Carole A. Mutzebaugh

Initially used to call together students and faculty to share religious or academic messages, convocations are used today in both colleges and academic units. Convocations can be used to open each semester's activities in any sized nursing program or college. A period of 2 to 3 years is required for the event to become "institutionalized."

This "calling together for a common purpose" provides an opportunity to communicate with nursing students, faculty, community nursing leaders, and others interested in nursing. Pre-nursing majors can be included to begin their association with the profession on-campus. Some schools may wish to invite family members or faculty from within the university.

A typical agenda includes introductions of faculty, preceptors, advisory committee members, student leaders from the National Student Nurses' Association, Sigma Theta Tau officers, and major nursing service representatives. Recognition is given to grant and scholarship recipients for community and professional service and accomplishments within the university community. An address by a local nursing leader is the highlight of the occasion. Alumnae or a student leader could also be selected as speaker.

Before adjournment, last minute course changes are announced or class information is clarified.

A reception before or following convocation provides socialization opportunities between students and practicing nurses. This can also become a time for hospital or military recruiters to share information with students. Reception sponsorship can be used as an additional recruitment aide.

Faculty development through the convocation program can range from planning the event for one semester or one year. Other faculty members or students can serve as program facilitators.

12

FACULTY INVOLVED IN ALL BUDGET PLANNING

Jacqueline Rose Hott

I don't know how long it really takes to feel like an *experienced* dean. I've been a dean for almost 3 years and an acting dean for a year before that. I am still learning and relearning. One of the major problems of deaning is the B-U-D-G-E-T. I have found that it is the well from which administrative power springs. When it's drying up, power decreases; when there's an increase (never a flood, but maybe a good rain), there is enough to give out rewards to keep thirsty faculty, staff, and students feeling healthier.

The innovation was to share the budget printouts at faculty meetings so that faculty would know how much there was in our specific well and how it related to the university's watershed. Faculty were included early in the next budget planning process. For example, they decided $1000 for subscriptions could be better allotted to support for conferences and that faculty would share magazine subscriptions among themselves. Instead of asking for a key to the supply closet or the copying machine so that the business director could supervise use of this equipment, faculty put their own limits on the numbers of copies they needed and supervised their own actions in a responsible, professional way. An ad hoc committee was set up to help the dean in setting criteria for special faculty development awards. Overall, faculty became more aware about how workload scheduling affected limited part-time/overload budgets. They responded with a task force to cut down on the amount of teaching contracts which had increased PT/OL and, instead, worked collaboratively to develop independent learning experiences for students, decreasing clinical costs without compromising the educational quality of the clinical program.

Educating and including faculty in the budgetary process can demythologize its mystique. It does not really cut down on the complaints but it does help the dean—and the faculty—to feel less isolated in dealing with that inexorable "bottom line."

13

SOCIALIZING AND PLANNING

Janice M. Stecchi

The faculty has found it extremely beneficial to meet together, once or twice a year, at a setting away from the department, with no agenda or planned business. Often teaching assignments or office locations prevent faculty from getting to know one another. It is amazing what a comfortable environment and nice food will do to help faculty members come together and plan joint academic and research endeavors.

14

FROM OPPOSITION TO CONCURRENCE

Barbara J. Barnum

In one of my early administrative positions, I inherited a faculty who had developed a long-standing tactic of factional blocking. Whatever one group wanted, another automatically did not. A situation arose when a National League for Nursing visit was fast approaching, with little constructive work in evidence. My tactic was primitive and dictatorial. I decreed that when any proposal was brought to the total group, the naysayers could not simply reject it but had to prepare an alternative plan instead—developed in equal detail.

It was amazing how soon they learned to respect each others' work—especially when the alternative was to redo the job themselves.

15

TO EAT AN ELEPHANT—ONE BITE AT A TIME

Margretta M. Styles

Life—and administration—are for me like eating an elephant; i.e., to be approached one bite at a time. When one operates under this philosophy, it is hard to single out one bite for special attention. However, I will share, not an innovation, but a fairly commonplace event, one of innumerable pleasant memories and feelings of accomplishment.

The first day I arrived full of enthusiasm at one university to assume the deanship, I was greeted by a minor uprising. Faculty and students were generally in an angry mood. A line of students waited at my office door to file a grievance. I soon learned that an ethnic minority student from a rural community had failed a critical nursing course in her junior year and was threatened with expulsion. Peers had rallied to her cause and were demanding that she be retained in the school. We sat in my conference room and talked for several hours. Later I met separately with the instructor involved. Finally we all joined together in a solution—probationary status and highly structured remedial support.

The student and I met several times as she continued through her extended program. After graduating, she would drop by to boast of her progress as a nurse and to request some occasional career counseling. We also discussed professional issues as she became a leader in the nurses' association and quite active in political affairs. Eventually she returned to the school for graduate study.

Surely an unremarkable story to submit for a treasury of deans' successes! However, when added up, these myriad "bites" of turning failure into success, negative energy into positive energy, and adversaries into friends constitute the sweetest rewards of more than 25 years in academic administration.

Part V

COMMUNITY COLLABORATION

16

OHIO ROUNDTABLE ON DECLINING ENROLLMENTS

Doris S. Edwards

When I became Dean of the School of Nursing at Capital University in August 1987, my chief concern was the steady decline in enrollments since 1983. Indeed, enrollments in nursing programs in Ohio had declined 27.1% during those same years. The appropriate response would need to extend broadly and involve diverse stakeholders and influencers. Consequently, we at Capital determined to host a statewide invitational roundtable discussion to identify further the dimensions and implications of the enrollment decline, to share strategies for promoting nursing careers, and to foster concerted and effective recruitment around the state.

Invitations to the Ohio Citizens League for Nursing, the Ohio Council on Nursing, the Ohio Department of Health Division of Nursing, the Ohio Hospital Association, the Ohio Nurses Association, and the Ohio School Counselors Association to co-sponsor the Capital roundtable with the School of Nursing were readily accepted.

The date of February 26, 1988 was selected and invitations were targeted at key nursing leaders in education and practice. High school counselors were included as well. Format for the day included a presentation of facts and figures by the Ohio Board of Nursing on the dimensions of the enrollment decline. This presentation, a chilling one, was followed by a panel discussion on the key influencing variables in education and practice. A successful model for recruitment, the Cleveland Nursing Now Project, was presented as a prototype for local community involvement.

The roundtable concluded with regional roundtable discussion groups on current and proposed local initiatives. The day ended with plenary discussion and group recommendations for the future.

Since the roundtable, a regional roundtable has been held in southeastern Ohio. Capital's local strategy was a fall nursing fair at a shopping mall, and this model is being implemented throughout the state as well.

Have we been successful? It's too soon to tell. We do know that this fall's (1988) enrollment decline was less than 1% over the previous year's figures. We are optimistic that the coming fall will show the downward trend reversed.

17

A NURSING EDUCATION ADMINISTRATIVE INNOVATION FROM A LIBERAL ARTS COLLEGE SETTING

Rosetta F. Sands

This—very personally satisfying—administrative innovation grew out of a commitment to foster collaborative relationships between our nursing program and hospitals in Northern New Jersey.

In the Fall of 1987, I received invitations to lunch from five of the vice presidents for nursing in the Northern New Jersey area. Each described similar concerns; all seemed to be associated with the nursing shortage. These were categorized as: reluctance of staff nurses to move from the primary nursing model to manager of care model; insufficient command of the nursing process, including health/physical assessment skills; and insufficient management training among head nurses, including delegatory skills. Each of the vice presidents believed our faculty could help them to alleviate most of these concerns, and asked that we share our resources with them.

While I was sensitive to the needs of each nurse executive and had a strong desire to help them, I knew the faculty resources could not be stretched to five different agencies. With only 14 full-time and 8 half-time faculty and a restrictive union contract, we were staffed to meet only the needs of our students. But I believed strongly that I had to figure out a way to help the five hospitals, involve the nursing education department in the delivery of nursing service, and maintain the goodwill of the faculty!

43

In a move to ease problems that had been described for me, I developed a model through which William Paterson College's Department of Nursing would form a consortium with the five area hospitals. The model would take advantage of the knowledge and skills of the nurse executives as well as the faculty. The model was presented to the nursing faculty and, after getting their approval, it was presented to the five nurse executives. The consortium agreement was signed by each participant.

The hospitals are Valley Hospital in Ridgewood, Chilton Memorial Hospital in Pompton Plains, Barnert Memorial Hospital in Paterson, the General Hospital Center in Passaic, and Wayne General Hospital. The nurse executives unanimously endorsed the model, and we believe it is the only model of collaboration among acute-care hospitals and a nursing program in a liberal arts college.

The consortium initiated a three-point program: to review and revise the categories of nursing service performed by registered nurses at the consortium hospitals, to provide advanced training in management to registered nurses in the consortium hospitals, and to enhance the pre-service clinical preparation of WPC's students of nursing.

The nursing faculty will work with the hospitals as needed as consultants to institute new models of health care delivery, delegating as many non-nursing functions as possible to hospital support staffs. This effort began with the onset of teaching of the nursing process and the use of nursing care plans at one of the hospitals.

The nursing faculty and the consortium hospitals have begun the preparation of hospital staff registered nurses to function as managers. Seminars in management and physical assessment for these nurses are being taught at WPC by WPC nursing department faculty, a team of nursing executives from the consortium hospitals, and myself. Adjunct faculty appointments were approved for each nurse executive teaching the seminars.

The third aspect of the consortium agreement focuses on the pre-service clinical training of baccalaureate students. Student nurses at WPC as well as other baccalaureate nursing students who have completed their sophomore or junior year will be offered three-credit summer clinical electives in which additional hospital clinical training will be obtained at the consortium hospitals. Their experiences will be under the guidance of WPC faculty and experienced nurse-mentors. This elective clinical experience is designed to refine developing skills of student nurses and improve their readiness to enter the rapidly-changing hospital practice environment. It is also designed to provide a pool of highly qualified applicants from which the hospitals can draw in the near future. Students enrolled in the clinical electives will be paid hourly salaries above the minimum wage. Faculty will receive summer contracts from William Paterson College based on union negotiated salaries.

Nursing executives from the consortium member hospitals who are working with me are Patricia Barrette, Director of Clinical Nursing at Valley Hospital; June Bowman, Vice President of Nursing at Chilton Memorial Hospital; Suzanne Latacz, Vice President for Nursing at Barnert Memorial Hospital; Gail Okiniewski, Director of Staff Development at the General Hospital Center; and Sandra Seigel, Vice President for Nursing at Wayne General Hospital.

18

A MODEL FOR LINKING FACULTY AND STUDENTS WITH CLINICAL ASSOCIATES

Jean Watson

I believe the best innovation I have made as dean was the creation of new clinical teaching-research models with University of Colorado clinical affiliates. During my first year as Dean of Nursing, I discovered the School of Nursing had a poor relationship with clinical agencies, yet the agency nurses and administrators were eager to have more formal, and informal, involvements and ties with the School of Nursing.

A series of collaborative models were established with different agencies that included the following:

1. Creation of Clinical Teaching Associate (CTA) positions among qualified professional staff nurses in clinical agencies to work with undergraduate students; the CTAs in turn are linked to lead faculty in the School of Nursing in the overall clinical teaching program; full curricular orientation and conferences and seminars are offered to CTAs from the different agencies. Special formal courses in clinical teaching, as well as other areas, are made available by the School of Nursing faculty as continuing education units (CEUs); CTAs receive 3 hours of free credit for School of Nursing courses; CTA teaching awards are given at convocation. Several CTAs have now completed advanced degrees in the School of Nursing as a result of these components of the collaborative model.

2. Creation of shared research positions with clinical affiliates, whereby a research faculty in the School of Nursing holds a dual position as Assistant Director for Research in a clinical agency. The researcher in turn offers staff development classes in research; facilitates and implements shared research programs and special projects; and fosters research and scholarship between and among faculty and students in the School of Nursing and professional nursing staff in the clinical agency.

3. Creation of Practitioner/Teacher (P/T) positions with clinical affiliates, whereby master's and doctoral level faculty function as unit-based experts, clinicians, and educators for students and for professional staff in the clinical agency. The Practitioner/Teacher helps to translate philosophy and theory of human caring into practice and educational activities in clinical agencies. The Practitioner/Teacher also helps to incorporate caring praxis dimensions into the academe and influence the nature of the nursing theory development and nursing research.

4. Creation of formal administrative links between School of Nursing and clinical agencies. The Director of Nursing holds the title of Assistant Dean for Clinical Affairs in the School of Nursing, and receives this appointment from the Regents of the University of Colorado.

Each component of the collaborative model better serves students, faculty, and clinical affiliates. The model helps merge value and philosophy; facilitates all three missions of the profession, i.e., education, research, and quality care; and formalizes institutional relationships and image of the university in the community and state. While the model emerged out of a need for improved relations, and with the goal to develop innovative approaches to link education, research, and practice and improve clinical teaching, it has generated a meta-effect and synergism that is beyond anything originally conceived of when first implemented. As a result, the activities keep growing and expanding into new models and projects for the future. Academic-clinical partnerships are now formed as an infrastructure for piloting new practice roles and restructuring professional nursing education and research that seek to improve health care in Colorado and the nation.

19

SIX SCHOOLS SHARE (AMICABLY) ALL THE COMMUNITY'S CLINICAL FACILITIES

Patty L. Hawken

One of the main responsibilities of an administrator is to facilitate the faculty's ability to teach, do research, and engage in scholarly activity. Faculty need to be relieved of many management activities. Too many faculty are involved in arranging clinical contracts, setting up media, scheduling classes and clinical times, and engaging in a myriad of other management activities that should be handled by administration.

When I first came to San Antonio, there were six schools of nursing: one each of diploma, AD, BSN, and BSN-MSN and two LVN schools. Each school would send faculty to all of the agencies and try to arrange for student clinical experience before the other schools could get there. The schools were in the habit of promising continuing education courses for the staff if they would allow that school of nursing access and student experience on the floors they wanted. The ante was increased yearly. When I arrived, some schools were devoting a half-time faculty position to inservice education for the hospitals and agencies in exchange for first choice student placement. The relationship between the schools was very tentative and wary.

One of my first actions was to meet with all the directors of the programs to discuss clinical placements. I proposed a clinical liaison system whereby each school identified one person to be the liaison person responsible for clinical assignments. In all schools this was an administrative person, not a faculty person.

The clinical liaison people arranged to meet three times a year prior to each semester, to go over each school's needs and to hammer out an agreeable plan among themselves for utilizing the agencies. Then each liaison person was responsible for dealing with one or two hospitals or agencies. The clinical liaison person would take the total requests to the hospital for the schools wanting to use that facility. Times, days of the week, the requested floors were all worked out in advance. The agency did not have to make decisions about which school should come. The agency did have final approval or disapproval over the plan and would deal with the assigned person. This system has worked well for 15 years. No school has circumvented the system and tried to do "side deals." The agencies like dealing with one person and not having to decide between schools. The schools benefit because they can work out clinical placements based on objectives and not who gets there first. It has also created a good working relationship among the schools and also a good working relationship with the agencies.

Within our School of Nursing the clinical liaison role is a full-time position, with the individual responsible for arranging all student placements (graduate and undergraduate); doing letters of agreements and contracts; exploring new facilities; checking out any complaints about facilities; giving each head nurse in every hospital or agency we use a copy of the appropriate student objectives, names of the students, dates and times of the clinical experience, and name of the faculty member. All these activities relieve the faculty of one more management task and allow them to spend time in what they have been hired to do—teach, do research, and engage in scholarly activity.

20

LEADERSHIP FOR PEACE

Anne Gudmundsen

Responding to a call to increase volunteers for the Peace Corps, I initiated contact with the Washington representative in order to explore the establishment of an agreement between the Texas Woman's University College of Nursing and the Peace Corps.

The first of its kind between a College of Nursing and the Peace Corps, the agreement calls for combining the course work for a graduate degree in nursing with 2 years experience in the Peace Corps.

The Peace Corps experience extends the College of Nursing's commitment to health promotion and disease prevention by providing an opportunity for the students and faculty to gain an international perspective about human needs for health care.

The continent chosen for this experience was Africa. The first student was assigned to Bonguel in the Gambia. She was trained as a midwife and is pursuing a doctoral degree at the Houston Center of the Texas Woman's University campus.

Working with a faculty member who had Peace Corps service and the students planning to study in Africa, I have developed a series of research questions to be answered over time. The longitudinal design will allow not only the identification of needs for care but also the opportunity to validate the nursing interventions selected for this population.

Currently, I am working with the Ford Foundation to secure funding to support student and faculty travel and research in selected portions of

50

Africa and to provide the dissemination of this knowledge through symposia and publications.

Because of my efforts to establish the agreement between the Texas Woman's University College of Nursing and the Peace Corps so as to explore a new infrastructure for health promotion and disease prevention on an international level, the Texas Woman's University College of Nursing received the Leadership for Peace Award on November 2, 1988.

21

SOLUTIONS FOR PROBLEMS OF ISOLATION ON A DELTA

Karen A. Saucier

Delta State University is located in a rural, isolated area of the Mississippi delta. Consequently, we often have problems with faculty recruitment. We are the only bachelor of science degree in nursing (BSN) program in at least 15 counties; another school offers an associate degree in nursing (ADN) program approximately 30 miles away to our east. The closest master's of science in nursing (MSN) degree is $2\frac{1}{2}$ hours away. The lack of proximity to graduate programs especially has resulted in a shortage of MSN nurses for faculty and in clinical preceptor positions for our students. Over the past 2 years, we have been fortunate to have created two innovative approaches to our shortages.

The first attempt came about when the director of the associate degree program and I became interested in developing an articulation agreement between our schools for RN to BSN degrees. Once we began exploring such an agreement, we both found that our needs were very similar. By sharing faculty when necessary (the director has a PhD as well), we could not only assist each other in faculty positions, but we could also increase each other's understanding about the different roles in nursing education. This has worked out quite well and has enthusiastic support from both administrations.

The second innovative approach actually was the result of student initiative. Several BSN/RNs approached a dean from another university in the state—one which offers an MSN in Community Health and Psychiatric Nursing—about establishing a satellite graduate program in the Delta. The dean and I met for dinner a month or so later and I indicated that I felt my administration would be very supportive of such a joint venture.

Although the process took several months to develop, partly because of difficulties at the state level of university administration, we admitted our first graduate students last August here in the Delta. The dean, one of my faculty, and I are teaching in the program. We anticipate that the director of the associate degree program will join us next year as a part-time faculty member as well. The degree will be conferred by the other university although we have had all classes and clinicals here in the Delta, utilizing Delta State University facilities. The program is flexible and meets four times a semester, nights and weekends. We have 19 students who we anticipate will graduate in May 1990.

We believe that we must be much more flexible and much less provincial in our thinking about meeting the educational and health needs of our state. If this program is an indication of such a change in thinking in our two schools, we are moving in the right direction.

22

MASTERS IN ADMINISTRATION—SERVICE AND EDUCATION

Barbara J. Barnum

The problem with most innovative ideas that come to my mind is that the most nifty ones soon become commonplace. The following, however, outlines an administrative team project; few good administrative decisions are insular.

The program involved establishing a first-class nurse executive program for busy, working nurse executives who wanted a nursing degree (master's or doctoral) and who had more cash than time. We created a program that cost an arm and a leg but provided all sorts of time-saving mechanisms. We provided services not available to the average student—preregistration, books already purchased, orientation weekends at a lush resort, library articles hand delivered, even rolls and coffee at the one-day-a-week intensive study.

We also made sure these students had the faculty superstars. The program was designed to be elite—from the best of classrooms to the best of teachers. (We succeeded so well that our students found the collateral courses from our prestigious school of business inferior by comparison.) The demands placed on the students, of course, were compensatorily challenging.

Most important, we defied all the rules about how learning takes place and offered the courses all within a single day of study. (To the loud objections of certain colleagues, I might add.)

Some college officers laughed when we proposed the program. They told us that nobody would pay such a price for an education, but we knew our target audience better. Needless to say, the program succeeded beyond our wildest dreams.

The hidden bonus was the cohort factor. Each group of women—strangely, a male student never applied—became a close-knit clan. Professionally, they still consult each other when problems arise in their working careers. The cohort factor enhanced the learning beyond our anticipations, more than compensating for the fact that the group didn't always become part of the larger university family.

We did, incidentally, do a lot of work to see that there were no jealousies and disaffections between the special program students and the regular program students within the nursing department. Students from both groups helped us solve the potential problems before they arose.

See E. Barba's dissertation (Teachers College, Columbia University) for details of the program. Such cohort programs are now offered in many more settings, but that was not the case when this program was designed.

23

PERSISTENCE PAYS

Jeanette Lancaster

When I came to Wright State University in 1984, I learned that the $80,000 which the hospital provided to the university on behalf of the collaborative agreement between the hospital's Division of Nursing and the university's School of Nursing was going to the University General Fund. Well, that hardly seemed fair since the School of Nursing did all the work to implement the collaborative agreement. During my first year, my limited efforts to gain the funds for nursing were unsuccessful. In year two, upon the appointment of a new president, I launched my campaign anew.

Since the university viewed itself as a metropolitan university which was closely associated with our partners in industry and because our faculty were not actively involved with the staff at the hospital, I requested that the money come to the School of Nursing to be used to support collaborative research. The funds were indeed transferred to nursing and now support a myriad of research efforts. Over 30% of the faculty, with their counterparts in service, are currently being funded to do research. The awards, while small, have greatly increased clinical research, collaboration, an *esprit de corps* among nurses in education and service, and feelings of worth among faculty.

One moral to this story is: Never assume that no will *always* mean no.

24

BSN SCHOLARSHIPS AND LOANS

Lillian R. Goodman

The very best innovation I have implemented as Chairperson of the Department of Nursing has been the creation of scholarship and loan assistance programs for baccalaureate nursing students. For the past year, I have worked closely with the chairman of the college Board of Trustees and with local hospital administrators in establishing the Worcester State College Collaborative in Nursing Education. Through the generous support of the chief executives of two private hospitals/medical centers, scholarships have been made available for junior and senior nursing students at Worcester State College. In addition, each of these institutions has made a commitment (4 years) to fund one faculty position. This allows the college to maintain the current enrollment level of nursing students during a time of fiscal crisis in the state.

I have also worked closely with a local philanthropist in obtaining tuition scholarships for five incoming freshman nursing students with the option for yearly renewal through senior year. This benefactor also provides tuition scholarships for registered nurse students.

25

VISIBILITY: "LIVING WELL WITH DR. PEGGY OPITZ"

Margaret (Peggy) G. Opitz

Increasing numbers of students today do not come directly from secondary education. These new students are "non-traditional," meaning someone who is not white, female, single, and 18 years of age. One way North Georgia College has used this information is to redesign our brochure, which now features a mature husband-and-wife student team. More important, we have taken our mature students to the air. A local radio station, WDGR, donated free air time as a community service. The station reaches 14 north Georgia counties, including the perimeter of Atlanta, and is owned and operated by a husband-and-wife team, the Andrews.

For our first broadcast, two enthusiastic LPN-RN mobility students were selected. A script was outlined and reviewed with them prior to air time. A half-hour time slot was determined with commercials and a song or two interspersed. The students, while nervous, performed well. They talked about how they selected the nursing program, the support they were receiving, the uniqueness of the program, the rich learning opportunities, and the rewards of nursing.

As department head, I provided background information concerning the nursing shortage and how the nursing department was addressing it, how we value nursing students, how listeners could obtain financial aid, and what the many benefits of being a nurse were. The outcome was better than anyone dreamed. The students became mini celebrities with their peers, applications were generated, and the nursing department increased its visibility.

An unexpected outcome was a request from the Andrews: Would I like to have a daily radio program? You can imagine my surprise! How could I say no when I thought of the benefits for nursing. Little did I realize the time involved. Yet this is offset by the opportunity to talk about any subject I desire. However, I do tell the Andrews in advance when I think a subject may generate controversy and we discuss it.

"Living Well with Dr. Peggy Opitz" has been broadcast for 18 months at this writing. The program airs Monday through Friday in a 5–8 minute time spot at 11:15 a.m. This is a peak listening time according to the station's market analysis. While I am at liberty to address any topic, my focus is usually twofold: (1) to enhance nursing's image and (2) to inform the public about health and nursing related issues.

It may be helpful to share the range of topics by the titles alone: "Halloween: How to deal with your fears"; "Why some people are luckier than others"; "Do you have the new spring glow?"; "How to put a new slipcover on your life"; "Maturity: The warm cookies and milk"; "How to play"; "How to really love your child"; "Anaphylaxis—that powerful reaction which can really kill"; "Do you want to be a hugger or huggee?"; and "Bridges—our links with others." The topics change weekly.

Periodically, the station also formally interviews me regarding pressing health care topics we, separately or collectively, have identified. I do enjoy being considered a nurse–health expert. Recent topics have included the RCT proposal and the nursing shortage.

Often, I get requests about topics people in the community wish to have discussed; they have then shared stories about how the information was helpful. Requests for scripts are frequently received. I always close each program with this line: "Be good to yourself and remember, as a nurse I care about you."

North Georgia College was founded in 1873, on the site of the former U.S. Gold Mint. I believe the nursing department has its own gold nugget with daily access to the air.

26

SCHOLARSHIPS AND THE NURSE SHORTAGE

Harriet R. Feldman

Although I have been in my position for less than 2 years, I would like to share an innovation (which has since sprung up elsewhere) that was implemented almost immediately after I began my employment at Fairleigh Dickinson University (FDU). In fact, the federal government has now adopted a similar initiative to address the nursing shortage.

During the early weeks of my appointment to the position of Chairperson of the Department of Nursing at FDU, I negotiated with two local hospitals for the provision of $10,000 merit scholarships to nursing students, with a contingency of work payback upon their becoming registered nurses. During the first year, a total of $90,000 was awarded to students with cumulative grade point average (CPGA) of 3.0 or higher in exchange for 2-year work commitments to their respective agencies.

Also innovative is the fact that the Agency Merit Scholarship contract has a clause naming the university responsible for retrieving any monies owed due to breach of contract. For example, if a student fails or withdraws from the program, FDU pursues them for the return of scholarship monies and guarantees replacement of the money or scholarship recipient to the agency. If the graduate leaves his or her other position after 1 year, the university provides a replacement (or returns the money) at no expense to the health care agency.

The Agency Merit Scholarship is one of the factors responsible for the doubling of enrollment in FDU's 1-year accelerated BSN program track for college graduates. Publicity about the scholarship, which pays most of the tuition for this program, has greatly increased the number of applications and enrolled students during the second year of scholarship awards.

27

A MODEL FOR
RESEARCH COORDINATION
COMMUNITY BASED

Crystal M. Lange

Saginaw Valley State University (SVSU) is a relatively small university with approximately 6,500 students, 140 full-time faculty with the university, and 14 full-time faculty in nursing. In addition, there is a faculty union which provides requirements related to teaching load and evaluation strategies. The university is located in a semi-rural setting which has a population base of approximately 500,000. There is no designated "medical center," although two hospital sites are regional centers for specialized services. Nine acute-care hospitals are in the area along with three public health departments with several home health providers.

NURSING RESEARCH

Quality client care is the ultimate goal of the nursing profession and is a concern of all nurses whether they are in education or clinical practice settings. Achievement of quality client care is facilitated by nursing research. All nurses can and should be involved in nursing research, directly or indirectly, as consumers or contributors, regardless of the setting. However, most settings have only portions of the necessary resources to carry out nursing research.

Involvement in research is more feasible through a collaborative effort in which resources are shared between and among education and practice settings. By means of collaboration nurses can draw upon the expertise of one another to achieve the mutual goal of improved quality of care through productive research studies. (See Figure 1.)

A collaborative effort produced a community consortium for nursing research in the region surrounding Saginaw Valley State University. The consortium is made up of the university, surrounding educational institutions, and area health care agencies. The group proposed and selected the consortium name: Research United for Nursing in East-Central Michigan (RUN-EM).

The office of nursing research is located in the College of Nursing and Allied Health Sciences at SVSU and serves as the regional coordinating

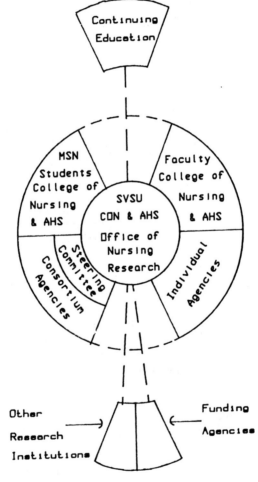

Fig. 1 A model for research coordination.

office to develop and maintain alliances for nursing research with the surrounding health care agencies. In addition, it serves as the coordinating office for research efforts of nursing faculty, students, and individual agencies. The research office maintains relationships with Continuing Education, other research institutions, and funding agencies. Representatives from the participating agencies serve as an ad hoc advisory committee. At least one meeting per year provides the opportunity for new agencies to become members. The office of nursing research is available to assist agencies with a self-assessment for membership. A university nursing faculty member is designated as the coordinator for the office of nursing research with limited released time each semester (the plan is to have it about the equivalent of one course or 3 credit hours).

The major purpose of the consortium is to encourage and facilitate nursing research while at the same time contributing to the maintenance of supportive relationships between and among the university and agency organizations. One of the advantages to SVSU is the support of action research efforts of both nursing faculty and graduate students. The advantage to the agency participants is the involvement of nurses in research activities and active participation in the network for sharing nursing research efforts in the region.

One of the outcomes of the collaboration is that nursing research which is practice-oriented is the vehicle for advancing nursing knowledge and influencing nursing practice. The research outcomes serve as the basis for clinical decision making and standards of practice. In addition, the use of current and relevant research findings as a standard for evaluation provides concrete evidence of quality nursing care.

The importance of practice-relevant research to the development and growth of nursing has been established (AAA, 1985; Rizzuto & Mitchell, 1988). Ventura et al. point out that effective nursing care leads to more cost-effective client/patient outcomes. Clients are more satisfied with the care and health outcomes when advanced nursing knowledge is utilized in nursing practice.

Murtha (1985) indicates nursing executives have an important role in supporting and facilitating the involvement of their staff in nursing research activities. There is continued need for research concerning the quality of care as it relates to the economic climate in health care today (Ventura et al.; Fagin, 1982). Specific care activities also need to be examined for cost effectiveness.

Agencies in East-Central Michigan have been marketing the area as a regional health care center. Nursing research is vital to the image of the area as a referral center. Within the agencies as well, the image of nursing is enhanced through nursing research activities. The research consortium provides the mechanism for sharing research expertise and resources. The arrangement increases cooperation among competing health care agencies, by allowing the collection of data on a larger scale than would be possible by a single agency and increasing the generalizability and usefulness of results.

Participation in the consortium requires the commitment to support nursing research efforts and to share in the communication network in the region. Consortium members are expected to follow the protocols/guidelines developed by and for the consortium. Agencies may select full or associate membership with annual renewal. A steering committee consists of seven agency members, one university appointed representative, and the nursing research coordinator who chairs the committee. Steering committee members serve 2-year staggered terms. (Annual fees for full members are currently $500; associate members, $100.)

Agency members receive newsletters and mailings, reduced registration fees for nursing research in continuing education programs, and participation in a minimum of one study annually. The research question is determined by a priority system with input from all agency members. Any member in the consortium may pose a problem for study. Agency members and associates may contract for a fee for consultation regarding a research project, tool design and production, instrument return and preparation, and computer analysis of data.

Authorship of articles is determined at the start of the research activity and can be negotiated if a change becomes necessary during the activity. Confidentiality is required and all members must subscribe to a confidentiality statement which assures that data will not be used to advocate or market an agency or berate others in the community.

In order to assist members of the consortium and members of the nursing community, the university provides continuing education regarding nursing research on a regular basis. Classes are offered on at least two levels, beginning and advanced, on a rotating basis. These offerings permit nurses to increase their knowledge base and become involved in clinical research activities in their respective organizations.

28

AN INNOVATION WITH LONG-TERM EFFECTS: "IF ONLY..."

Norma M. Lang

Early in my years as dean, I began to hear discussions of how the problem of nursing could be solved if only.... The "if only" would be followed by some description of what nursing service leaders should do if the spokesperson was from a nursing education leader; and in reverse, if the speaker was a nursing service leader, the "if only" would be followed by a description of what nursing education leaders should do. I believed these discussions to be nonproductive and thought about what we might do together.

The chancellor of the university and I decided to host a luncheon for chief executive officers of hospitals from the major metropolitan area, in the chancellor's conference room. We were pleased with the number who came to discuss what we might do together to improve nursing practice and nursing education. We also were pleased with the positive exchange of information, concerns, and suggestions.

The process of the meeting provided a chance to jointly renew a commitment to nursing. The positive ideas generated provided many open doors for rapid implementation of several activities. Subsequent meetings with vice presidents for nursing continued the momentum.

Several examples of the major ideas generated that day were implemented, and still serve as well including:

• Research contracts with hospitals that enabled faculty to carry out research jointly with clinical nurse specialists, nurse administrators, and other nurses in practice

- Successful joint pursuit of endowed faculty research chairs and funding for nursing research
- Funding of elective enhancement courses for undergraduate students, ensuring a higher level of acute-care nursing skills
- Establishment of clinical preceptors for senior undergraduate nursing students
- Joint clinical practice and teaching appointments

A luncheon may not be considered a very innovative activity, but the open communication between university and nursing educators and chief executive officers and vice presidents is innovative and necessary on a continuing basis. Pointing a finger and saying "if only" is not useful; talking together about what we can do together will provide us with many more creative opportunities to improve the quality of nursing practice and nursing education.

29

PROMOTING LINKAGES

Sue T. Hegyvary

The greatest challenge facing a new dean is "getting the lay of the land" to see what activities and directions are appropriate. The assessment of "fit" with the environment is essential. This idea certainly is not original, nor is it a specific "innovation" in my 3 years in the deanship at the University of Washington. Yet if I try to describe my most important and central activity, I think this is it.

In assuming this new position, it appeared true enough to be trite that I needed to link the past and present with the future. During a strategic planning effort in the first year, the weight of that activity became apparent. My role as dean would be to lead into the future an excellent school with top ranking nationally, with excellent research programs in an outstanding university, and with comprehensive educational programs. Was it positioned for continued excellence or for resting on its laurels and stagnating? How was it perceived in the surrounding community, in the state, in the region, nationally, internationally? With excellence in research and education, what about practice and promotion of the overall goals of the profession?

Faculty expressed many views of strengths and deficits but were able to center on some immediate priorities. Within the following year, we planned, approved, and implemented the AD-MN program for registered nurses desiring to pursue specialty education. Giving attention to the registered nurse population opened the door for linkages with the 18 community colleges in the state that provide associate degree nursing education. It also gave a message about valuing clinical practice. Many other activities devoted to strengthening relationships among research, education, and practice continue to occur as a result.

In another environment, the programmatic outcome may have been different, but the guiding principle of linkages likely would have been the same. The assessment of appropriate linkages is an ongoing activity that determines the future of relationships and indeed the future of success of any school. It also gives a great sense of challenge and excitement to the deanship as a role of leadership in a constantly changing environment.

Part VI

CURRICULUM

30

WHEN IN DOUBT DIVERSIFY

Judith A. Balcerski

For 25 years the Barry University School of Nursing had been a traditional baccalaureate program admitting high school graduates at the freshman level with the first clinical nursing course in the sophomore year. No more. Today we have three master's programs and five options leading to the baccalaureate degree. The undergraduate course sequencing plan on my office wall looks like the bus schedule for New York City. Students are delighted with the choices, even if they are at first confused.

The traditional undergraduate 4-year pattern still exists (Basic Option) but to meet emerging needs four other undergraduate options were added one at a time to the present mix. Taken separately, these five options are clear and discreet. Taken together, they make an intricate pattern of movement hopefully reflecting grace, not chaos.

The RN to BSN Option was added first. RN students are older and have more learning experience than traditional students. They require courses reflecting their adult learning needs for different content, teaching methods, clinical experiences, and course schedules. Thus was created a flexible evening program responding to the needs of this group of students which are quite different from those in the Basic Option.

Next we responded to the student who wanted to change careers and to earn a second bachelor degree. Students in this group want to complete their program as quickly as possible and long days of classes are accept- able tradeoffs to ensure a short program completion time. Thus the

12-month Accelerated Option was created. In this option liberal arts requirements are completed first and nursing last, in contrast with the Basic Option where both are taken together. Accelerated nursing courses are taken in 5-week blocks as compared with the 10-week blocks for the Basic and RN and BSN Options. This option is physically and intellectually demanding but strongly preferred by graduates.

It then became clear that the Basic Option was not structured to respond to the transfer student who presents 60 credits of applicable liberal arts credit but who does not want to take six academic semesters to complete the nursing courses. By combining parts of the Basic and Accelerated Options, students are able to complete the program in four academic semesters and the intervening summer. We created the Two Year Transfer Option. Completion of this option in five semesters instead of six, saves the student one semester of private university tuition and enables the student to graduate one full year sooner than the old pattern. Clearly the Two Year Transfer Option pleases transfer students.

The fifth option is the newly designed LPN to BSN Option. As with the RN student, nonduplication of content is our objective. Although competency demonstration and mainstreaming is the current plan, a separate track of lower division nursing courses is anticipated for the near future.

Advising students of their options is critical to the smooth operation of our program. Students are able to change from one option to another as necessary and appropriate. Tracking of individuals is essential. As a result of our creativity in manipulating the basic factor of time, we are able to please most of the students most of the time and student satisfaction is our reward.

31

TWO NEEDS SERVED: HEALTH CARE FOR THE COMMUNITY AND GRADUATE EDUCATION FOR NURSES

Ildaura Murillo-Rohde

As Dean of the College of Nursing, State University of New York, Downstate Medical Center in Brooklyn, I immediately raised salaries for the faculty who badly needed more money, and guided them to required doctoral degrees for professorial rank, promotion, and tenure. Also I restructured the program to eliminate summer classes for students and faculty.

My main objective was to establish a Graduate Program, something my predecessors had been trying to develop for 15 years but had never realized. I became dean in April 1982, and by May 1985 we had a Graduate Program approved by the state university authorities and the State Education Department in Albany. We also obtained a training grant for $458,294 for 3 years from the nursing division in Washington. This amount of money was rather unusual at that time.

Since I had no extra funds to develop the Graduate Program, I had to use one professor and myself during one semester. I had appointed a Graduate Program Committee to give us ideas and review our drafts. I also brought in a few consultants to help us with format and to shape our ideas in the best possible way. Brooklyn and Queens did not have a Nursing Graduate Program and the nursing community was in great need of one. Since New York City has a number of colleges and universities with the regular and usual programs, I thought that for our program to be accepted and not opposed by surrounding colleges and universities, it had to be different and innovative, to meet a need that had not been addressed by other programs.

With the advent of diagnosis related groups, very sick patients were being discharged to be cared for at home. Nurses were mainly responsible for such care. The community health nurse had not been prepared to assume this new role. I felt there was need to prepare a clinical nurse who could fill the gap between hospital acute care and rather intensive home care. The faculty and Graduate Program Committee agreed with my idea and we set to work. We developed a program in "Continuity of Care for Adults in Urban Settings." The president of the medical center was very pleased, the people in Albany were excited, and the program was approved without any problems.

We sent our training grant proposal to Washington, and not only was it approved and funded for an unusual amount for the time but it was also welcomed with, "there was need for this futuristic new master's program." The program started in 1986 and is doing very well. Other specialties are being added to the initial one. Graduates of the program are in demand by community agencies, and the graduates feel their education prepared them for their much needed work in the community and home. In addition, the graduates can meet requirements for nurse practitioners.

32

ACCELERATED MASTERS FOR NURSE EXECUTIVES

Barbara J. Barnum

It seemed foolish to educate nursing practice administrators and nursing education administrators separately, in their own little worlds, continuing the crazy tradition of two disparate camps. My faculty and I thought the two should learn to talk to each other rather than point fingers of blame. And that meant that they had to develop an understanding of where the other guy came from.

We started small—with one course in which the students were mixed in approximately even numbers. The first class meeting revealed the usual adversarial positions of service versus faculty, faculty versus service. Then we selected administrative topics for the course: personnel, budget, quality assurance, staffing—you name it. We looked at each subject as it was enacted and lived on each "side."

Sometimes it was enlightening to assign students to prepare presentations from the other side. It was a great way to lay bare the false preconceptions of each group. More often, they simply failed to consider the contextual differences of their mates' environments.

You can imagine what an exciting class a topic like quality control would create. How did quality control of nursing practice differ from quality control of teaching, for example? What were the limitations and problems in each setting? What were the opportunities? Could good teaching really be measured? What did the principle of tenure do to quality? How did mixed versus professional staffing affect quality in a practice setting?

Could patient—or student—outcome serve as an effective measure of quality input? Mostly, our students learned that principles didn't exist in a vacuum; they had to be applied in diverse, specific environments, each with its own characteristics.

The students loved the course and each side learned to appreciate the difficulties, challenges, and rewards of the other domain. Several took jobs in the other side over the summer to gain greater appreciation for the differences that so often divide us.

Once the faculty had developed and tested a few joint courses, we devised a program that mixed would-be executives from both settings. They had some courses together, some apart of necessity. A lively course of study, you'd better believe. With luck, our future leaders will have the wisdom and the understanding created by such an endeavor—the ability to see nursing as a united profession.

33

ADVANCED NURSING PROGRAM IN PLACE—*NOW* DEVELOP A BASIC PROGRAM

Donna Diers

The very first implemented innovation I ever did was to memorize the budget for my initial discussion with the Deputy Provost. Although he was stunned by the level of detail I had mastered, this isn't a very exciting story.

Although I did not propose our innovative 3-year master's program for college graduates, I did lead in its implementation. My predecessor, Margaret Arnstein, had marshalled the program through the university approval system, and had she lived, she would have chaired the implementation. As it was, she died in October of the first of two planning years, and it was left up to me.

The major problem, it seemed to me, was that outside of our own undergraduate experiences, our ignorance of modern basic nursing education was considerable. The Yale School of Nursing had been entirely a graduate program for 15 years or so, and we simply had no foundation upon which to build. We were creating a bottom to a structure that already had a top. Oh, we had lots of opinions about how other people had done basic education wrong, but how to do it right?

In retrospect, that ignorance, including my own, probably worked to our advantage. We did not have years of having toiled in the integrated curriculum versus medical model vineyards to overcome, and while we have various prejudices, that's about all they were. The major curriculum planning breakthrough came in a painful faculty meeting when the faculty

77

were resisting having to teach basic nursing, when they were all specialized. First, the late Vivian Romoff, a psychiatric nurse, spoke suggesting
that the faculty simply teach what they were already good at—such a
simple solution hadn't occurred to any of us. Then Katherine Nuckolls,
head of our pediatric nursing program, proposed that the specialist faculty
approach the curriculum design task by thinking about what knowledge or
experience the advanced curriculum expected of students entering it.
Since both of these contributions recognized what the faculty felt was
being lost—their knowledge of their special fields—there were great sighs
of relief, and, almost overnight, a curriculum was developed.

We had to notice the nervousness of the faculty over whether we would
be able to stuff in our students' heads everything they were ever going to
have to know, fast, in the 1 calendar year that was dedicated to the basic
experience. At one point, there was a move to bring the students in a
month early and give them all the basic nursing techniques and skills in a
blitz. I was moved to inquire about whose problem this was solving—ours
or the students'—and the suggestion died.

We had to invent everything, from admission application forms through
curriculum, uniforms (we decided not to have one), ceremonial occasions,
administrative structure, to say nothing of budget. The most important
initial decision made (and I made it, alone) was not to eliminate the
existing regular master's program, but rather to let the new one hang
under it, absorbing the college graduate students into the regular specialty
programs after their initial basic year. Among other things, that meant a
much more secure financial base, since the federal funds upon which we
already depended were intended for graduate preparation of people who
were already nurses.

All kinds of issues surfaced, even before the first students did. An
application to the first class came in from a man in prison. We found out
what he was in prison for: rape. The enrolled master's students staged a
small uprising: they weren't going to serve as "big sisters" for these people
who were going to have it so easy. We had planned a very heavy science
course, but by July before the first students were due to arrive in September, there was still no one to teach it. A gift from heaven, one Linda
Dublin, with a PhD in neuroscience, arrived with her post-doc husband,
granted a late fellowship to Yale. We had no extra money to open the
program except a little siphoned off from the alumnae fund to support the
science position. In December, Santa Claus arrived early with Kellogg
Foundation support. The State Board of Nurse Examiners had to be
convinced to approve 2 years of a 3-year curriculum; the university had to
be convinced to grant a certificate attesting to completion of the program.
The latter was easy. The former took the intervention of an alumna who
was the night supervisor for the person who chaired the state board. She
poured advice and coffee into the chair, and her attitude changed.

The first class arrived, scared to death, nearly as scared as the faculty. And then the second, third, fourth, and on and on. The program not only survives, it prospers to this day, producing unusual and fascinating women and men nurses. It's become a model for nursing for college graduate programs. It has reformed our institution and made connections for us throughout the university we would not otherwise have had.

Funny thing is, as a faculty member, I had voted against it in the first place. As dean, I got the credit.

34

THE MSN: EDUCATION IN ANESTHESIA FOR NURSES

Patricia A. Chamings

An innovation of which I am proud has been the merging of an existing certificate anesthesia program into the School of Nursing and offering a Master of Science in Nursing (MSN) degree. The anesthesia program took some time to implement, but the faculty in the School of Nursing and the anesthesia faculty worked on developing the curriculum so that both groups felt ownership and respect. (For further information, see *Journal of Nursing and Health Care*, May 1989.) The curriculum meets all the criteria for accreditation for both National League for Nursing (NLN) and the Council on Accreditation, American Association of Nurse Anesthetists (AANA) and is really reconceptualized for a graduate program. Many more applicants than can be accepted apply each year. This *is* an excellent program of which we are extremely proud.

35

VANDERBILT UNIVERSITY SCHOOL OF NURSING'S "BRIDGE" TO THE FUTURE

Colleen Conway-Welch

In 1985 the Vanderbilt faculty and I ventured down a risky road, making a major programmatic change to phase out our bachelor of science in nursing (BSN) degree, which had 50 years of excellence and tradition behind it. However, the school was moving into its eighth decade of existence and facing declining BSN applications and budget problems. Dramatic changes were needed to position the school for a continued leadership role in nursing education in this country.

Since 1985 the school has undergone a radical curriculum reorganization in order to create the "Bridge" program, which enables students who have not already earned a BSN degree to enter the master of science in nursing program. The three-semester Bridge contains the traditional undergraduate "generalist" nursing content. After completing the generalist nursing courses, students enter into the three-semester specialist nursing courses.

The Bridge program is based on the belief that the first professional degree in nursing should be based on in-depth knowledge of liberal arts and science, should be specialty-related, and should be offered at the post-baccalaureate (or graduate) level. The increase in knowledge and scope of nursing responsibilities as well as changes in roles, functions, and practice settings require a graduate nursing education which draws from a rich undergraduate liberal arts and science education *and* a baccalaureate degree in nursing or its *equivalent*.

Due to the present diversity in nursing programs and future applicants, educational opportunities must be made available to facilitate progression to the master's degree as the first professional degree. The Bridge program was designed to provide multiple entry options to the MSN for students who may be associate degree or diploma nurses or non-nurses with a college degree or at least 72 hours of undergraduate coursework. The program, based on a variety of cognitive styles, life experiences, and professional backgrounds, allows all students to achieve the same terminal objective.

The Bridge program has attracted over 30,000 inquiries nationally and internationally in the 3 years of its existence. The program attracts students with a wide variety of educational backgrounds and life experiences. The average age of our students is 34 years with an age range of 21–67 years! Students enter the program with associate, baccalaureate, master's, and doctoral degrees. Many of them are entering nursing as a second career. This diversity of student body enhances the quality of the educational program and I believe it will be enriching to the discipline of nursing as well.

The nation's health care system is moving through a revolutionary period requiring dramatic changes in the organization and delivery of health care. A similarly dramatic change is required in the education and training of health care professionals. The US Department of Health and Human Services projects the minimum number of master's prepared nurses needed will exceed the available supply by 295% in 1990 and by 334% by the year 2000.

Vanderbilt has positioned itself to meet this urgent need by producing master's prepared nurses who are educated to give direct care to complex patients with complex needs.

Vanderbilt's innovative Bridge program is an effort to address the need for well-educated nurses who can fill a variety of advanced practice roles as we enter the 21st century. Vanderbilt graduates are prepared to respond quickly and enthusiastically to the changing demands of our health care delivery systems of today and tomorrow.

I consider the Bridge program to be the most exciting innovation I have implemented in my 5 years as Dean of the School of Nursing, and I am very grateful to Dr. Jean Watson, Dean of the School of Nursing, University of Colorado, for being the catalyst for my early frustration which directed my thoughts to the need for a Bridge into nursing education. It has been my privilege to have the faculty interest and administrative support necessary to undertake such a dramatic change in the direction of the school. It is my hope that Vanderbilt's Bridge program will become a model for nursing education of the future.

Part VII

SUPPORTING/ENCOURAGING FACULTY

36

THE DEAN ENCOURAGES, SUPPORTS, HELPS IMPLEMENT

Margaret L. Shetland

I have been writing my response in my head ever since reading the invitation and seem to focus on one idea: that, of the many valuable and imaginative innovations that were implemented during my tenure as Dean at Wayne State University, I do not take credit for one. I think about the Center for Nursing Research, primarily you and Virginia Cleland; the Nursing Home Project, you and Maria Phaneuf; the Health Care Clinician Project, Dawn Zagornik; the TV Teaching Program, Rhoda Bowen; the Program for Mothers of Abused Children, Lorene Fischer and Marjorie Fields; the Committee on Racial Awareness, Lorene Fischer; the Nurse Clinician and Intensive Care Projects at Detroit General Hospital, Irene Beland, Kathlene Monahan, Lucy Brand, and others; and many more. I did steer the faculty in curriculum revisions in the development of curriculums based on nursing theory and goals, and a realistic program for registered nurse students.

As I reflect on this experience, I realize that my administrative style, which I hoped would encourage creativity, was based on Chester Barnard's *Functions of the Executive*, which I studied at the Maxwell School at Syracuse University. His idea was that authority rests with the person who actually performs the functions. This notion leaves the executive with the functions of supporting, encouraging, and helping to implement ideas emanating from those in the front line. My administrative style also had origins in the work of Dwight Waldo and Kenneth Benne, which I developed and used in Teaching Supervision and Administration. As faculty knew, sometimes I was successful in applying these concepts and sometimes I failed.

37

QUALIFIED FACULTY

Geraldene Felton

University culture demands publications and research as the benchmarks of a productive academic. Getting to be dean requires an understanding of what is going on around you. Indeed, nursing deans need that quality since the survival of the college is at stake. And survival is more and more dependent on the reputation associated with good management skills, broad pragmatism, and effectiveness in a job that is much more complicated than ever before. Central administration expects the dean to provide direction and to exhibit the courage to stand up for what the school really is good at. Meeting this expectation requires being able to make sound, deliberate choices and sticking to them, keeping an eye on the larger goal while adjusting when need be to altered circumstances along the way. Above all, it requires being principled and confident.

When I arrived at my present position, tenure decisions had just been made about 22 nursing faculty. Some were tenured as assistant professors. Some were promoted to associate professor (inappropriately). We had to clean up our academic ranks, move nondoctorally prepared faculty out of the tenure track, and set criteria—so that no one became assistant professor without the earned doctorate.

The dean must find ways to maintain a sense of direction and a concern for the future of the organization. Such sense and direction requires knowledge of the enterprise as well as enthusiasm and positiveness about the future. Among ways I do this are exchanges with counterparts at conferences and seminars, identifying role models, pinpointing areas for improvement, and taking blocks of time to reflect on the state of the enterprise. Such reflection asks such questions as: "Where are we going? Where should we be going and why? What principles are we using to get there? In what ways are my efforts enhancing or impeding the vitality of the enterprise?"

Personnel decisions are both painful and ambiguous. However, with the support of my boss, the vice president for academic affairs, and the president of the university, in 2 years we were able to eliminate procedural weaknesses and adopt new policies for required qualifications for appointment, retention, promotion, and tenure; move most nondoctorally prepared faculty to lecturer (nontenure track) positions; demand more faculty research and scholarly productivity; and nurture the ethos of scholarship, in addition to emphasizing excellence in teaching. Now, all newly hired assistant professors already have the earned doctorate. In a faculty of 80, only 6 associate professors (out of 17) and 5 assistant professors (out of 30) are not appropriately credentialed. In 1989, we are more productive than ever, have more internally and externally funded research, more dedication to teaching, and more and better relationships among our academic colleagues and our nursing service colleagues. We have found that the college is nothing more or less than the sum of its people and their collective commitment to competence and creating a vibrant and lively environment, and their willpower and energy in accomplishing the school's mission.

38

FACULTY SHARE DECISION MAKING

Mary E. Conway

This approach to one aspect of administration which I shall attempt to describe here may not legitimately fit the definition of innovation. However, for me, in terms of my personal growth as an academic administrator, it *was* an innovation and in the setting in which I applied it, it was almost revolutionary.

I accepted my second appointment as a dean in a school of nursing in a college where collegial self-governance was honored in name only. It was not so much that self-governance was frowned upon but rather that the culture of the institution for years had been one of paternalism and one in which ideas new to that culture, or somewhat deviant, rarely got further than a polite one-time hearing. The culture in which I found myself probably was not unique but its impact on me was profound. I had come from an institution of higher education where faculty were consulted on almost everything new that was proposed, or subject to change, and where intense debates were the norm. Faculty's approval or disapproval of the administration's initiatives was often the determining factor in whether a proposed policy was adopted. Thus, by contrast, faculty in the "second" school seemed apathetic. For example, a question put forth by me for discussion at a faculty meeting early in my tenure—whether a faculty merit evaluation plan should be put into place—met with almost no response. It is hard to think of an issue which might be expected to generate more debate among college faculty than that one. It caused me to do some reflection.

My innovation, if it could be called that, was a conscious decision on my part to refrain from making *any* decision in which faculty might be affected or about which they might be even remotely concerned. In carrying out this decision, there were times when uncontroversial questions or issues were raised about which the dean might conceivably render a decision and be fairly certain there would be no adverse response from faculty. However, I believed that if my self-imposed strategy were to be successful, I would have to be consistent in refraining from making unilateral decisions. Was this a strategy to avoid criticism or accountability? Absolutely not. Was it a strategy that would delay or impede the "work" of faculty and others? The answer is no. A strongly held belief underlay this strategy. I believe that only when those persons who are the key actors in an enterprise have an intense, personal investment in it can that enterprise have a hope of achieving excellence. And a large part of that personal investment involves each individual's dealing with issues, taking reasoned positions, and considering possible outcomes for alternative actions.

Donald Walker (1979) makes a similar point regarding the administrator's role in decision making in academia. He said, "Administrators should not use the existence of a participative style of decision making as an excuse to evade responsibility themselves. That's not the point of the style. The aim is to get better decisions, more effectively made." He goes on to say that one must not give up too soon and "fall back" on problem solving from the top down.

I was tempted on several occasions to do exactly what Walker cautions against—falling back on problem solving from the top down. But the temptation was short-lived.

For a few months, participation by faculty in debating academic or all-college policy was limited. Very few faculty were willing to be risk takers in a situation which (as they perceived it) might be fraught with peril. That is, faculty under a previous dean had made it a practice to determine what the dean's opinion about a particular issue was before rendering any independent advice or opinion. Their usual role was to second or affirm the dean's stance. It was not long, however, before role expectations for the dean on the part of faculty, and those for faculty on the part of the dean, were substantially altered. It became clear through actions taken at both departmental and general faculty levels that faculty, in general, had reconceptualized their role and had taken on ownership of the academic enterprise. And while it would be inaccurate to ascribe any singular cause and effect relationship to the decision that preceded this alteration in the culture, concomitant developments were increased respect between faculty and students and greater satisfaction on the part of students with their academic programs.

REFERENCE

Walker, D. (1979). *The effective administrator*. San Francisco: Jossey-Bass, p. 189.

39

CURRICULUM—A FACULTY RESPONSIBILITY: THE MSN FOR RNs

Patricia T. Castiglia

For the associate dean responsible for academic affairs, important functions include analysis of the curriculum, nursing needs assessment, and planning for the future. Change, however, can be difficult even when people realize that there is a need for change. An administrator who understands the social change process can help to facilitate needed change.

One of the most difficult changes to implement at SUNY/Buffalo was the opening of the master's program option to registered nurse students. Faculty generally believed and were committed to the baccalaureate for entry into the profession. About 8 years ago, a special curriculum for non-BS nurses was instituted. This action was taken in response to the needs of large numbers of non-BS prepared RNs in this area. When the issue of the possibility of an RN to MS program was addressed, faculty were generally reluctant, at first, to even consider such a program.

Some faculty members felt that offering the BS option was sufficient in terms of our resources; others remained committed to the necessity for baccalaureate preparation. Still other faculty members saw no advantage in terms of requirements for the degree, that is, the curriculum could not be adjusted. Yet other faculty felt that the integrity of both the baccalaureate and master's programs would be threatened. A small number of faculty and administration felt that selected RN students might benefit from the opportunity to move toward their career goals in a more efficient manner. They pointed out that a number of RNs returning to school were returning for the BS in order to progress professionally in a particular specialization area. In fact, these students usually went on for the MS degree right away.

Faculty were at an impasse about what to do. Curriculum is a faculty responsibility and administrators need to proceed cautiously when offering curriculum suggestions. It took 2 years for the faculty to establish an "honors-type" program for RNs which enabled selected RNs to begin master's level coursework prior to completing the BS. This was accomplished through the formation of a task group composed of both graduate and undergraduate faculty. Actually very little substantive work was accomplished the first year. A trial period was instituted during which undergraduate RNs could take approved graduate courses as electives or as courses not to be applied to the baccalaureate degree. The committee spent most of the time focusing on the curricula of both programs, on community needs, and on their own feelings. In the second year, however, the committee was directed that a decision must be made. The committee made a recommendation to all faculty that RN students meeting the criteria for admission to the graduate program be encouraged to take a sequence of courses identified by the committee. The recommendation was accepted and implementation is in its second year. Although the program currently implemented does not completely meet the need for an accelerated program for RNs, it has provided the pilot or perhaps a first phase of implementation which can be evaluated.

This situation is an example of a program innovative in this geographic area. It provides an example of a need that administration recognized and endorsed but certainly would not implement by administrative decree. Faculty participation, adequate time allocation for discussion, informational resources, and a willingness to let faculty truly decide a curriculum issue were the key administrative components.

40

INNOVATION OR PLANNED DEVELOPMENT?: FACULTY DEVELOPMENT AND FINANCIAL RESOURCES

Rosalee C. Yeaworth

Franklin P. Jones is given credit for the quote, "Originality is the art of concealing your sources." As with originality, innovation seldom materializes as something totally new or as the work of a single person. I came to a school that had sound programs, using the latest technology to provide an off-campus baccalaureate program for RNs, and an extension division in Lincoln. The master's program in nursing and the nursing research center were furthering graduate education efforts.

As dean, I believed my mandate was to provide leadership to develop further the research and scholarly productivity of the faculty and to continue to meet the most pressing nursing educational needs of the state despite decreased federal funds and a flat state budget. Toward the first goal, I developed the "faculty assistance for doctoral study" policy which allowed faculty to qualify for half salary for a year of doctoral study. We recruited a director of the Nursing Research Center who came with a federally funded project. We hired a full-time person to provide faculty with assistance in research design and data analysis and a half-time person to assist with computers. Secretarial assistance was provided for typing grants and manuscripts. Financial support was provided for travel to present research and for covering the cost of slides and posters. Additional necessary space for laboratory or research staff and merit increases were made available to those who succeeded in getting federal funding. In line with the Medical Center, the College of Nursing developed a supplemental salary policy to permit additional money to people who had part of their state salary replaced by grants. To allow for recruiting the best qualified persons possible when lines opened and to permit existing faculty to have the opportunity to teach graduate courses as they developed their credentials, the college was reorganized by departments.

In trying to keep nursing education accessible, we resisted a recommendation to close our Lincoln Division to save money. With encouragement from the legislature, we worked with a regional hospital and its diploma nursing program to develop a division of the college in Scottsbluff. We are in the process of planning to make our master's program available in sites other than Omaha.

The research and scholarly thrust has moved external funding from an internal seed grant of a $2000 American Nurses' Foundation grant to the current year's $750,000 in external research funds. For the past 4 years, the college has qualified for a biomedical research support grant, and we have submitted a proposal for a specialized center grant. Faculty success rates are high on publications and presentations at regional, national, and international research meetings. Our proposal for a PhD in Nursing has been approved at the Medical Center level and is now under review by the all university graduate council.

There has been much ongoing change in the college in the 10 years I have been dean. Yet there is little I can claim as "my innovation." I have worked with faculty and higher administration to continue a developmental process congruent with professional nursing today.

41

FACULTY CHALLENGED
TO EXCELLENCE

Grace H. Chickadonz

In the state of Ohio, there was a program to foster selective excellence in higher education. Schools competed for the awards on the basis of excellence already achieved, then specified how the money would be used to extend that excellence. This was a very positive program in that the application was written about the school's strengths.

I got the idea of duplicating the excellence model within the School of Nursing at the Medical College of Ohio. A significant part of the award was designated for faculty projects. These were to be selected on the basis of an internal competition, just as the school was competing for the overall award.

Faculty were encouraged to develop their ideas for special innovations and to spell out their needs for accomplishing them. Projects were to be selected on the basis of quality and value toward meeting the school's goals.

How exciting it was when we won the award and were able to implement the innovation. Some very creative products emerged from the faculty's proposals. Innovations in teaching were the most common projects such as videotaped interviews with nursing leaders, computer assisted instruction, and special guest lectures on nursing and history which were also videotaped.

Not only did the project contribute new innovations for the school, the process created pride and enthusiasm in the school and the faculty.

42

ADMINISTRATION AS EVOLUTION

Nan B. Hechenberger

You are right that there is hardly a nursing publication today that doesn't report some valuable ideas and programs from the University of Maryland School of Nursing. The vast majority of these, however, are not my ideas but the ideas of an incredibly competent, professional, and dedicated faculty. I suppose the part that I play here is that I allow faculty to implement their ideas with a good deal of freedom. I am a firm believer in hiring the best person for a position and then leaving that person alone to do what you hired the person to do. I suppose the major contribution that I make to the University of Maryland School of Nursing has to do with my administrative style. It is to delegate and hold accountable; it is to respect the dignity and integrity of each individual; it is to confront conflict and to do so in an honest and straightforward manner; and to be fair and even-handed in making administrative decisions.

Our administrative process here is one of organization development. It is an ongoing process that has resulted in major structural and curricular changes—our master plan for program evaluation, our faculty workload system, our strategic plan for the School of Nursing, and an integrated system for public relations, marketing, and fund raising. I suppose one thing that is innovative here at Maryland is that we try to get the most "bang for the buck" out of anything that we develop. We have marketed both our Master Plan for Program Evaluation and our Faculty Workload System to the public and have raised about $78,000 through sales of these products. We have developed two grant funded special projects related to measurement and evaluation and have published two books based on outcomes of those special projects. The copyrights and royalties from these books have been signed over to the School of Nursing. In other words, we try to develop a program around any particular product we develop. We have a project approved now that will be related to strategic planning, marketing, and evaluation. We believe that we have something to offer here at the University of Maryland and we are anxious to share some of our successes with the rest of the nursing community. I think we have been particularly successful in doing that.

These are the kinds of things from an administrative perspective that I would share with you from the University of Maryland.

43

"ACRES OF DIAMONDS"

Phyllis Drennan

Every day I try to remember "one never steps in the same river twice." The author of this quote is an anonymous ancient Greek philosopher. The quote helps me to focus on the future, while at the same time to use present and past experiences wisely.

A dean has the opportunity and obligation to create opportunities for others. This inspiration came from Russell Conwell's remarkable classic essay, "Acres of Diamonds": "an opportunity abounds in every yard, in every city, on every farm, if only you study that opportunity and create it yourself." As a dean, I try to create opportunities for our faculty, our students, our friends, and our alumni; there are acres of diamonds in our own schools and universities.

44

TRANSPOSING A DREAM INTO REALITY

Carol J. Gray

A dean always has opportunity for creativity. Whatever the circumstances, the key to transposing a dream or vision into reality is quite simple. Set your sights, chart the course, be invulnerable to cross currents and alligators, and surround yourself with exceptional individuals who share the same dream and who will stay the course.

Although I have not heard Dean Brown use these words, I know she must share a common philosophy. She has been, after all, an extraordinary role model.

Part VIII

OPENING / CLOSING / PROMOTING PROGRAMS

45

FACULTY CAN TEACH, PRACTICE, AND CONDUCT RESEARCH

Marie L. O'Koren

There was renewed excitement and enthusiasm among the faculty at the University of Alabama in Birmingham School of Nursing as a release time quarter plan was initiated. Some faculty who often taught the same course content for four consecutive quarters and others who suffered from "burnout" eagerly anticipated relief from their monotonous schedules and looked forward to a change of pace and an opportunity to increase their participation in clinical practice, improve research productivity, and other scholarly pursuits.

Since all faculty are on a 12-month appointment, the plan provides for three quarters each year to be devoted to assigned instructional activities and the fourth to an option of either research, writing, clinical practice, enrolling for additional formal education, or a combination of two or more of the options. During some years a faculty member may have the release time quarter in the fall and in subsequent years in the winter, spring, or summer quarters. Every attempt is made to maintain flexibility in the plan to accommodate the needs of the faculty. For example, it is conceivable that two consecutive release time quarters might be taken to complete a project.

The release quarter plan is applicable to all full-time faculty who hold the rank of instructor or above. New faculty are eligible for participation after at least four quarters of employment.

Individual faculty inform their level chairman of the plan for the option chosen and seek approval for the release quarter 6 months in advance of that quarter. The level chairman, in turn, submits a comprehensive time schedule plan for all faculty to the appropriate assistant dean who then forwards it to the dean. Faculty stipulate specific plans for the option to the level chairman prior to the beginning of the release time quarter. The plan includes objectives, activities to be undertaken, and the anticipated impact on either the faculty member, the situation in which the project is to take place, the level or the school. A final productivity report is submitted by the faculty member to the level chairman at the end of the quarter and the reports are forwarded to the respective assistant deans and to the dean. The evaluation of the plan is based on data contained in the specific faculty plans and the final productivity reports.

The plan resulted in increased faculty productivity, further faculty development, improved clinical expertise, and improved relationships with nursing service as a result of the faculty's working with the nursing staff on a day to day basis in delivering nursing care.

Additionally, faculty are able to meet tenure and promotion criteria with greater facility than they did in the past, inasmuch as they are provided a specific time segment in which to carry out activities related to tenure and promotion. The plan also led to a more manageable categorization of faculty activities and, therefore, was more conducive toward establishing equitable faculty work loads.

Finally, it must be acknowledged that a plan of this nature could not have been implemented without the support and encouragement of the University of Alabama in Birmingham administration and the administration and staff of the university hospitals. We are most appreciative for the assistance given to us in gaining additional faculty positions, making arrangements for faculty practice and research, and in helping to identify additional resources for the success of the plan.

46

GOING AGAINST THE STREAM

June Leifson

As a new dean, still overwhelmed with the unknowns of the position, I was faced with a university decision that had been made and announced, but had not been accepted by the majority of the faculty and student body. The decision was to discontinue the nursing program located 50 miles from the main campus. The nursing program was to be consolidated, not reduced. We were given 2 years to plan and implement the task.

The Rationale: The students needed a strong general education and the full opportunity of a university experience. It was the belief that a university experience should be more than courses, lectures, clinical experience, concerts, and plays. These activities alone do not constitute the entire intellectual environment of the university, although they are part of the university environment. Association and discussion with serious students from other disciplines and the more extended encounters with faculty members not in their own major were felt to be important parts of the university experience. Of greater importance yet in the university was the environment of faith in the church-sponsored university. An occasional visit to campus did not substitute for the experience a strong student had in being immersed in the university environment.

Problem Solving: All impact factors were identified and studied. The factors identified were the lead time needed, transportation costs for students and faculty living in the area, notification and public relations problems, supportive courses that would be needed on campus, class-

103

rooms, conference rooms, office spaces, parking concerns, clinical laboratory facilities and, most important of all, attitude change.

Change Agents: Since a number of the faculty lived in the area and the move would impact them, they were asked to form a committee to define the problems and to develop possible solutions.

Students: The students would continue to use the clinical facilities in the area. Classes and competency laboratory would be on the university campus. Orientation to the move was announced immediately to give the students time to become aware of the change. Students in the program were allowed to finish their program where they were located. All new students were told before entering the program they would be located on campus for all classes and labs. Group meetings were held for all the students, plus letters were sent to all pre-nursing students.

Attitude: The greatest problem was changing attitudes. In responding to a petition signed by 72 students requesting reconsideration of the move decision, it was noted that attitude change is impossible with some, moderate with many, and accepted by few. The 12 faculty involved also had difficulty with an attitude of acceptance. One faculty member retired, the others have moved to their offices and facilities on the main campus.

Outcome: The majority of the students and faculty are immersed in a university setting. The move has been made with a mixture of feeling: most accepted it with some reservation, a few with great pain, and a few with satisfaction. A number of the graduate faculty feel they have lost potential students due to the move. One exception to the original plan was made. Two courses are being taught in the extended area due to special guest faculty teaching the courses.

Change can be made: It is not without pain, joy, and satisfaction.

47

RESEARCH COLLEGE OF NURSING: A NEW COLLEGE, A NEW BSN PROGRAM

Barbara A. Clemence

In 1985, I accepted the challenge of my dreams: establishing a college and a new baccalaureate nursing program. In February 1987, the North Central Association of Colleges and Schools accredited Research College of Nursing as a college. On October 18, 1988, Research College of Nursing was accredited by the National League for Nursing. A new college and an innovative joint nursing program without Rockhurst College was viable and blessed by the accreditors.

Students receive a joint bachelor of science in nursing from Rockhurst College and Research College of Nursing. Strong, effective, and caring linkages are in place among students, faculty, and administrators of both colleges. Our students study on both campuses all 4 years and continue their community service, social activities, and friendships on each campus as well. Faculties from each campus co-teach in the liberal core and nursing electives courses. Faculty and students participate through committees in the governance of both colleges.

This accomplishment is a capstone experience of my nursing career. The venture has been a great growth experience for me personally, and also for students and faculty. I have used my accumulated knowledge and skills to influence political pressures on college development; to gain trust of the governing board of the college and the administrators of Rockhurst; to challenge and guide faculty in program development; and to enable RCN faculty to grow in knowledge and instruction in baccalaureate education.

My greatest pleasure and reward is the growth of the nursing faculty who are now engaged with enthusiasm in research and in a variety of scholarly endeavors to maintain their teaching excellence and give leadership to the profession. For me, Research College of Nursing is a dream which became reality.

48

A SCHOOL'S AUTONOMY

Enid Goldberg

Many things have occurred during the almost 17 years that I have served as Dean at the University of Pittsburgh School of Nursing. I am sure that the majority of these events can be replicated in many other schools.

Many individuals are aware that from 1985 to 1989, the School of Nursing was under tremendous pressure to merge with the Schools of the Health Related Professions and Pharmacy. I believe I provided the leadership to faculty to ensure that the school remain autonomous as it has been since its development in 1939. This was a very difficult period of time, and I learned a great deal from it. Individuals are not too interested in mergers; therefore, some constituencies did not offer much assistance. Closure of a school is very dramatic and raises many emotions. The concept of the merger was approved by the Board of Trustees, but the school continued to fight for its individual existence. I am sure that there are individuals within our system who were of great assistance to the school and I will never know who they are.

The message to be gained is that if you believe in something, you must use all your energies to protect it. The issue was finally resolved in our favor in November 1987.

49

"CHAIRPERSON'S CHALLENGE": CLOSE THE NURSING PROGRAM

Barbara F. Haus

Eight months after my election to Chairperson of the Albright College Department of Nursing, I found myself face to face with a proposal from the college administration to close the nursing program using a process meant to take less than a few short weeks to complete.

The situation I faced was overwhelming and seemingly hopeless. Enrollments had declined, expenses were increasing, and the college was moving toward a greater emphasis on the liberal arts. Nursing, in the eyes of many, was not central to the mission of the institution.

To stop the closure, immediate action was needed. My response to the college committee which addressed the issue of program closure seemed futile. Time was needed, and it was not available. *But* the nursing students, showing their ability to rally around a cause and take a risk, carried out a sit-in demonstration in the college library. Their demand to have the item of voting on nursing program closure removed from the college faculty meeting agenda was met.

Letters and phone calls poured in to the college president and the Board of Trustees protesting program closure. Support from alumnae, nursing colleagues, physicians, and the community was overwhelming. My energy to fight the proposed closure was renewed and over the summer I gathered the data necessary to plead my case.

Declining enrollment, finances, and the place of nursing in the small liberal arts college had to be addressed in such a manner that faculty, administration, and trustees would be convinced that program closure should not occur.

I countered the concerns about declining enrollment with information regarding increasing salaries for nurses, improved funding for nursing education, new recruitment strategies, and nationwide efforts to change the image of nursing.

In conjunction with an economic professor, an analysis of the cost of the program using projected revenues and expenses was conducted, and I was able to demonstrate that the program required a minimum of 36 full time equivalencies (FTEs) to meet expenses.

Finally, I argued that nursing personifies the liberal arts. I asked where else in the college could students have the opportunity to learn to apply the natural and physical sciences, social sciences, humanities, and fine arts in actual encounters with their fellows? Yes, I said, nursing might not seem essential to the college, but the nursing students' contribution to courses outside their concentration, based on their far-ranging and broad exposures to the diverse groups in the population, would be noticably absent if the program was discontinued. I stated my belief that nursing was an integral part of the college and sorely needed to achieve diversity.

In the fall of 1988, the college president and I addressed nursing program discontinuance before the faculty. My contentions were found to be worthwhile, and the faculty voted to keep the program open. Later, the Board of Trustees followed suit. My coup was accomplished, and the battle was won. I did not emerge unscathed but, hopefully, am wiser and stronger for the experience. May my experience benefit those who come behind me to continue the struggles that nursing and nursing education face in the decade ahead.

50

FROM DEPARTMENT TO SCHOOL OF NURSING

Rita M. Carty

As a nursing student and later as a faculty member, I always jokingly said, "When I have my own school, this is what I'll do." Never in my wildest dreams did I ever believe that one day I would have "my own school." In 1981, I was selected through a national search as Chairman of the Department of Nursing at George Mason University; I was the second chair of this new nursing program and followed the program's founder, who was a very charismatic leader. Those were big shoes to fill, and I decided the best thing to do was not to try to fill them but to try to make footsteps of my own.

Of course, it took at least 1 year to figure out what was going on in the program and university. As time sped along, I fulfilled the role of chairman in the university and functioned as a dean in regard to the community, profession, and nursing organizations. A study I conducted of schools of nursing as compared to departments or divisions of nursing clearly indicated that schools had more resources, including faculty and budget; achieved more external funding; and had an almost exclusive hold on elected members to national organizations, including officers and committee members. At the same time, changes in the university were occurring that provided a window of opportunity for reorganization and the possibility of achieving school of nursing status for the program.

My strategy for pursuing this goal included asking professional colleagues to write and express their support for a school. I also sought support from health care agencies in the community where our students received their clinical experience and asked nursing alumni to express their support through calls and letters. An impressive response and show of support was received. The president of the university, although somewhat taken aback, responded to every call and letter he received.

There was some internal opposition to my plans. This opposition came in large part from the Chair of the Faculty Senate and was based on his idea of what he thought the university should look like as it grew and developed. Nursing alumni called his office on a continual basis, which provoked him to tell me to "call off my dogs." Fortunately for nursing, the president of the university did not agree with him. He is now a mathematics professor.

In 1985, the Department of Nursing became the School of Nursing at George Mason University. Although there was no way of predicting what would happen to me if school status was attained, I fortunately was named the first dean of the School of Nursing in 1985. I happily remain in this position today.

Part IX

UNITING PRACTICE AND EDUCATION

51

A CHAIN OF INNOVATIONS

Dorothy M. Smith

In my opinion, my very best innovation was my assumption of two titles at the time of my employment in January 1956 at the University of Florida as it started a new program in nursing—namely Dean, College of Nursing and Chief of Nursing Practice at our teaching hospital, which opened on campus in 1958. This innovation—a combined role for nursing education and practice fairly common at one time in our history—was unpopular in 1956. But for us, this one innovation acted as base and impetus which spawned new and exciting procedures and policies during the next 17 years. For example:

1. Development of the unit manager system as a function of hospital management, not a part of nursing.
2. Inclusion of the hospital administrator as a member of the Health Center Council with the deans.
3. Delegation of authority as well as responsibility to the unit (ward) representatives of medicine, nursing, and hospital administration (decentralized authority.)
4. Development of patient care teams involving nursing and medical faculty, nurses, medical residents, and medical and nursing students (and members of health related professions as required).

5. Development of a systematic approach to the identification and solution of patient nursing problems. This required the development of data collection tools and methods of record keeping as well as methods of problem solving.

6. Storage of nursing records as a part of patient charts for availability for research and learning. (In most places nursing records were discarded.)

7. Faculty practice (clinical) and the involvement of hospital employed nurses in teaching became valued conditions of employment.

8. Decentralization of authority and responsibility to academic sections (departments) for the quality of practice, teaching, and research relative to the section. Section members included undergraduate and graduate faculty and hospital employed nurses.

9. Assignment of students to patients for professional care as and when needed (not just 9–12 a.m. or 7–10 p.m.).

10. The combined role provided for a nursing practice viewpoint on administrative and academic committees.

11. Development of standards of nursing care related to disease and medical treatment as well as standards related to the nursing care of the *patient* who has the disease.

All these sub-innovations were born, nurtured, and grew, but for various reasons they were not institutionalized in a sufficiently solid manner to last over time with the inevitable personnel changes. They required an enormous amount of energy and commitment (though not necessarily of time) because their survival required constant and consistent communication at all levels within professions and between professionals. We flourished as a bright gem when our health center was small. With increasing numbers of patients, students, and medical specialists as well as decreased funding, our innovations were not strongly enough entrenched to withstand the push from both medicine and nursing toward more traditional and separate functioning. Our innovations fundamentally of a collegial and decentralized nature with emphasis on the growth and development of patients, staff, faculty, and students were seen as unaffordable luxuries—yet, according to Florence Nightingale in "Notes On Nursing," fresh air, cleanliness, and nutritious food were all, in her time, considered luxuries in patient care.

52

THE FULL INTEGRATION OF PRACTICE AND EDUCATION IN NURSING

Luther Christman

The notion of the full integration of practice and education is not a new or novel concept. Professions such as dentistry, human medicine, veterinary medicine, and clinical psychology have produced many excellent versions of the concept. Integration models have not been implemented in the nursing profession in an analogous fashion. The full integration at Rush University called for service and education to be under the management of one person with the title of Dean/Vice President for Nursing. This integration was reinforced at the Associate Dean/Vice President for Nursing level. Each of the two associate deans had approximately half of the service responsibility. In addition, one associate dean administered the undergraduate program and the other the graduate. The next level of integration was at each chairperson level, where the dual accountability was particularized to a specific clinical area. The faculty members, in their roles as practitioner/teachers in each specialty area, became the linchpins that held the system together through their practice and teaching. Thus, questions about student placement and rotation could be resolved quickly and with relative ease.

Several benefits were derived from this model. The role socialization of students was facilitated because the practicing faculty members were very aware of the nursing care plan of each patient assigned to students. This enabled students and faculty members to focus primarily on the key scientific and clinical issues for each respective patient. Students went to

117

the practicing faculty for their clinical experiences instead of faculty taking students to the unit as guests or visitors. The staff viewed students as junior colleagues instead of persons impeding the work effort of the units. Because of the economy of effort in having students share in the care of their patients, the faculty members could give more individual attention to students while enabling them to round out the professional role. Furthermore, the curriculum could be maintained with more relevance to the changing world of care. Finally, a more accurate evaluation of students could be done as well as a more perceptive evaluation of faculty members by students.

The staff nurses profited by the consistent and regular presence of the faculty as caregivers. The faculty members were on the units when the students were not there. This enabled staff nurses to secure consultation about practice issues; to have inservice educators readily available; to benefit from the rapid, regular, and accurate dissemination of new knowledge; and to be stimulated to enroll in graduate programs. Self-governance of the professional staff had beginnings similar to those of the faculty.

The clinical graduate programs, especially the clinical doctorate, could flourish in this milieu. Not only were skilled nurse practitioners available but the easy communication between physicians, and other members of the health team, enlarged the graduate students' insights into clinical care and clinical research. All the specialties could be offered.

Clinical research could be done with less stress and frustration. The basic issue of good research is asking the correct question. The daily confrontation with clinical problems helped in sorting out the burning questions. Furthermore, the presence of practicing faculty collaborating closely with physicians in care endeavors made access to patients a relatively untroubled pathway.

The financial resources were mobilized more effectively. The service budget was about seven times the size of that for education. The combination of these two into one whole made it possible to support 280 faculty members. Other advantages accrued by having a large total budget that had flexibility. The rich mixture of this number of faculty integrated fully into the staff produced a high quality of nursing care. Thus the students, at all levels, could experience and participate in seeing how patients could prosper when nursing care was of a high order. Their professional and ethical predispositions to act could be strengthened and their growing edges stimulated. All parts of the system supported each other.

53

A SAGA IN SOCIAL CHANGE

Loretta C. Ford

In 1972, I was recruited to the University of Rochester in the dual position of Dean of the School of Nursing and Director of Nursing in Strong Memorial Hospital (the university's hospital) to implement an organizational design to unify nursing practice, education, and research. For the next 14 years, implementation of the model occupied the interest, intellect, and energy of a large team of nurse leaders who fulfilled multiple roles as leaders, scholars, teachers, and clinicians. This team worked cooperatively within nursing and collaboratively with physicians, hospital administrators, and others. The team goals were to professionalize nurses in practice, to advance and expand excellence in the nursing education programs, and to improve practice and delivery of nursing service through scientific investigations. Through the efforts of the many people involved in this great social transformation of nursing, many salutory changes occurred.

The education programs were expanded from the offering of a baccalaureate program through doctoral and post-doctoral research. Nursing Practice grew to an almost full professional nurse staff with a clinical advancement system, participation of nurses in hospital governance, faculty practice and joint practice, committees and models of practice with physicians, nurse practitioners in ambulatory and inpatient services, clinical practice research projects, and a host of other innovations. Faculty gained in strength, stature, and sophistication in their research efforts as independent investigators of nursing phenomena. The years were filled with blood, sweat, tears, and lots of successes on the part of many committed nurses.

Our frustrations stemmed from the lack of the kinds and numbers of leaders and scholars needed for a dynamic system that had many uncertainties in the beginning years. Many senior faculty leaders in other schools were either unqualified for our needs or unwilling to risk the changes required to unifying practice, education, and research in two disparate nursing systems of education and research. Recruitment was difficult. Too few people realized that system change is basically social change and a decade of effort is a very short time in which to realize results. Many nurses are politically naive and tend to function mainly on a personal basis vis-à-vis employing political strategies.

As nursing gained solidarity across education and practice, other power brokers felt some alarm and were threatened by the power base the unity in nursing was building. The reallocation of resources demanded and the shared power won by nurses created uneasiness in other professions and administrators. Over the years, the regulatory and financial environment changed and institutions struggled for external resources and autonomy to maintain the quality and expansion of their endeavors. Shortages of nurses have added to the difficulties the hospital faces today. Additionally, universities face similar constraints and problems. Albeit, one would hope that the philosophy, values, and structure built into the unification of nursing practice, education, and research will not be lost as stresses and strains of the system experience the ebb and flow of societal changes.

For myself, the implementation and many successful outcomes achieved could not have been possible without the group of committed, competent, creative, and courageous nurse leaders who served as associate deans, clinical chiefs, academic chairs, faculty clinicians, and practitioners, and a host of other leaders in medicine and hospital administration with whom we worked and fought and finally became loving critics of each other.

54

"A RESIDENCY PROGRAM"

Gladys Sorensen

Residencies for newly graduated nurses have been bandied about for years, with many nursing leaders denigrating the idea, viewing it as cheap labor from new graduates. The term *resident* was used in this project since it was meaningful to the funding source. At the University of Arizona, the state appropriates educational funds through the College of Medicine to University Hospital for salaries of residents for service to the hospital and teaching of medical students.

In 1984, I decided the College of Nursing would seek funds for newly graduated master's students for a year or two of guided experience in teaching and in some aspect of service. These learners would contribute to the college and to the hospital. Salaries offered would be slightly less than that paid to a beginning instructor with a master's degree. (Later we adjusted salaries upward.) The hospital administrator of nursing favored the idea, provided her budget was not used.

The Chief Executive Officer of the hospital approved and granted the College of Nursing $96,000 of the residency funds to initiate the program.

RESIDENCY

Flyers advertising the residencies indicated this was an opportunity for newly graduated, fairly inexperienced master's prepared nurses to learn teaching with an experienced faculty member as mentor and one or two of four aspects of nursing service with a mentor from University Hospital nursing staff. The residents' time was to be divided approximately equally between education and service. The four areas from which nursing service could be selected were: advanced clinical nursing, management with a head nurse, staff development, or research. A resident could change the service emphasis, if desired, every 6 months but needed to maintain the teaching aspect. The mentors were provided at no cost to the program. The service portion was in the same clinical area as the teaching. We started with three residents, two in medical-surgical and one in child nursing.

The resident shared a clinical group of students with faculty the first semester and carried a group on his or her own after that. In some instances, the resident supervised a clinical group of students the first semester with guidance from faculty.

Since residents were considered learners, sessions were held with them to discuss activities and offer guidance. Mentors evaluated residents each 6-month period. Residents evaluated the program and made suggestions for adjustments.

Maximum length of the residency is 2 years.

INTERNS

An unanticipated added benefit was sufficient funds available for selected baccalaureate students to serve as interns in University Hospital for 8–10 weeks during summer. Undergraduate students in the past were hired as nurse aides, with limits on what they were allowed to do. By enrolling for independent study, they were classified as students and permitted to carry out activities they had been taught as students. They must have completed two of the five semesters in the nursing program before becoming interns.

The nursing residents and nursing service personnel supervised the undergraduates during the internship. Conferences with students were held to discuss patients and their care. Evaluations were conducted at summer's end by all involved.

OUTCOMES

Residents, interns, faculty, and service personnel, for the most part, felt the program was a success. Funding has been increased somewhat and today, 1989, the program is still in existence. One article describing the residency has been published by two residents, and one presentation has been made to a national group.

Part X

NURSES ASSOCIATIONS

55

MEMBERSHIP FOR THE TOTAL STUDENT BODY

Enid Goldberg

On a light note, I have always had some dreams regarding our undergraduate student body organization. For many years, actually since its development, the school has had a strong undergraduate student group with officers, etc. As the years went by, I was able to provide the students with a faculty member who was actively involved with the American Nurses' Association. She was able to organize a small group of students as members of the Student Nurses' Association of Pennsylvania (SNAP); however, that did not solve all our problems. The non-members of SNAP were five times as large and when they went to the university student government for financial resources, they always received a very large sum of money. The majority of the money was utilized for nonprofessional activities. Finally this past year, the faculty member has been able to organize our entire undergraduate body of over 500 students to become one student association and all of them will be members of the Student Nurses' Association of Pennsylvania. This has indeed made me very happy.

Along the same lighter lines, we had a ceremony called Black Banding. At the beginning of the fall term, junior students received a quarter band and senior students received a full band. I have always believed that this was strongly related to practices in diploma education. The event became more meaningful when we provided scholarships and awards to students at this affair. However, this year the student body has decided to change their uniforms and in addition they made the decision not to wear caps. Students are going to receive bars as have our male students in the past and we will no longer have a Black Banding ceremony.

56

GROUP MEMBERSHIP PIQUES INTEREST AND PROMOTES INVOLVEMENT

Marguerite J. Schaefer

The time was 1966. Stirrings of major student unrest had surfaced on many university campuses including the University of Pittsburgh. Students in the School of Nursing were especially vulnerable since the school had just passed through a difficult period in its history. As a new dean, I felt that it was incumbent on me to find a way to defuse a potentially difficult situation.

In 1966, there was no effective undergraduate student organization in our school, no clear channel for communication between students and faculty administration except for individual student academic counseling done by faculty members. No one was responsible for student affairs. Students were telling us in many ways that they wanted more attention and a "piece of the action."

Even though my knowledge of organizations and the practice of management was minimal at that point, I believed that students were consumers of our product, namely, nursing education. As such, we needed to listen to them and we both needed structures that encouraged dialogue. Further, I believed that students, most of whom would work in organization, would profit from direct participation in an organization and opportunities to exercise leadership roles.

Plans for structures to encourage dialogue and student participation included creating a new position to be known as Assistant Dean for Student Activities and a student organization. All student affairs including academic counseling were assigned to the office of the assistant dean. Among other responsibilities, it was expected that the assistant dean would serve as a role model and teacher in helping students to identify and resolve organizational problems associated with their lives as student nurses. The new dean was to become a member of the school's Administrative Committee made up of department chairpersons in order to provide the necessary linkage to academic administration. Additionally, students were to be organized by classes, each with their own elected officers and representation on a school-wide Student Nursing Organization.

The plan was partially implemented in the first year of my deanship and became a fullfledged reality 1 year later. The results were as hoped for. We weathered the late sixties and early seventies with flying colors. Students were not only enthusiastic about their organization and the opportunities it afforded but also reported that their experience as members was an integral part of their education.

From the perspective of 23 years, the implemented plan reported above was not terribly innovative but it was new for us. More important, it was an innovation that exemplified sound administrative practices. First, feedback from consumers was recognized as important to the success of our enterprise. Second, a structure was created to support a piece of our work which we deemed important and without which the work would have proceeded slowly, if at all!

57

"A COURAGEOUS AND TIMELY ACT"

Rozella M. Schlotfeldt

It was in the 1960s that much recognition was given to the fact that discrimination against women was widespread in employment and other areas in the United States. The Civil Rights Act of 1964 was amended, and in 1972 the Equal Employment Act was passed and the Equal Employment Opportunity Commission (EEOC) established; the latter revised the code of federal regulations and established guidelines with a view toward having practices comply with the law. State EEOCs were established to investigate, conciliate, and negotiate complaints in their respective states. Failing in those efforts, complaints led to civil suits.

In February 1972, the American Nurses' Association (ANA), having investigated the retirement benefit practices of the Teachers' Insurance and Annuity Association and College Retirement Equities Fund (TIAA-CREF) noted that monthly retirement benefits paid to women were smaller than those paid to men of the same age even though accumulations in their individual accounts (premiums paid) were the same. The justification given by TIAA-CREF for the practice of using sex-biased tables was that men, on average, live less long than do women. At the same time, retirement benefits paid to black TIAA-CREF beneficiaries who, on average, also live less long than do white men, received no such compensatory increments in their monthly retirement checks. The ANA then sought volunteers among its members who would be willing to file complaints with their respective EEOCs against the management of TIAA-CREF for violating EEOC guidelines. The ANA officers were

128

willing to file the complaints and suits, if necessary. Along with two other nurses, I signed the necessary complaint, but not before I advised my (then) university president in writing that the ANA would file a complaint on my behalf and that the university, through which TIAA-CREF retirement plans were provided, would also be named and was potentially subject to suit.

Since the university president had already named an equal opportunity agent and made known his wish to eliminate evidence of discrimination within the university (I had previously sent his agent numerous evidences of discrimination within the university), I included this paragraph in my communication to the president:

> Knowing your wish to eliminate such discriminatory practices, I assume that you would favor and encourage women faculty members here to file complaints. I would appreciate having your reaction.

His response indicated that he would not "oppose or disfavor." I signed the charge of discrimination, convinced that it was the right thing to do. My grandmother taught me well by virtue of her often quoted colloquial expression, "Right will out!" I have typically been guided by it. Surely I am convinced that leaders must have courage as well as conviction in order to implement needed changes.

On August 18, 1973, the ANA sent out a news release that the EEOC had ruled that there was "reasonable cause to believe" that the use of two separate (female/male) actuarial tables to calculate university faculty benefits was in violation of the Civil Rights Act of 1964 and the Equal Employment Act of 1972. That decision resulted from a complaint filed by ANA on behalf of one of the nurses in whose state EEOC acted reasonably promptly and was "expected to have national implications" (ANA news release, August 18, 1973). Quite understandably, local newspapers carried items about the ANA's complaints on behalf of three (named) nurses who originally filed complaints.

In November 1973, I attended a social function attended also by a member of our university's Board of Trustees and his wife. Both had previously been very friendly, but on that occasion, the board member ignored me. When I spoke with his wife, I questioned this apparent change in her husband's attitude and, not having received a plausible justification, sought an appropriate time to question the person who so obviously was angry with me. Thereupon he vented his anger directly at one (me) who had so badly treated the university (the "most despicable thing that it has ever experienced"). It was quite obvious to me after our conversation that he knew many circumstances of the EEOC complaint except the fact it was filed with the knowledge and sanction of our university president. I then apprised him of that fact, adding that it surprised me that he *could* think I had acted without the president's knowledge and sanction. When his shock was obvious, I quietly told him that I would apprise the president about our conversation. The following day I put a brief account of the discussion in a letter to the president from which I quote:

> When I realized that Mr.———might not appreciate that collaborative efforts of administrators and faculty members toward their common goal . . . , I told him that I had, of course, cleared with you before participating.

I then gave the president a brief update on the complaint and ended the letter thusly:

> It is to be hoped that a resolution will emerge from the conference, conciliation, and persuasion now ongoing and that our efforts will have been consequential with regard to elimination of discrimination that none of us condones.

The president promptly replied to acknowledge my letter, with thanks.

Subsequent to ANA's original request, other nurses joined in the effort and finally the ANA's complaints were filed on behalf of nine nurse faculty members in several states to demonstrate that the problem was widespread. Although all those complaints were decided in favor of ANA, the TIAA-CREF did not change its practices until a New York federal district judge ruled in favor of a plaintiff in that state who used the TIAA-CREF's reluctance to reach agreement with ANA as evidence for that court's ruling. In the interim, other women's groups had taken action on behalf of their members and the suit was settled on behalf of one of those complainants.

Since I had retired in July 1982, I was the only one of the three original ANA complainants who received a lump-sum payment from TIAA-CREF in compensation for the amount I would have received, had I been a man. I wrote to both of my colleagues (both still active) to apprise them of the amount I received because I knew that the consequences of our action would never be so dramatically made evident to them as it was to me.

In April 1985, under a front page headline, "Women, ANA Win! Teachers' Pension Checks Now Equal," a reporter told the story from which I quote:

> Much of the credit for this step toward pension equity for women goes to nine nurse faculty members who were willing to challenge the system, and to ANA for supporting them. (The American Nurse, *11*(4) April, 1985.)

Right will out!

Part XI

ALUMNI AND PUBLIC RELATIONS

58

CELEBRATION, INVOLVEMENT, AND PUBLIC RELATIONS

Maryanne E. Roehm

The Indiana State University School of Nursing celebrated its Silver Jubilee during the 1988 calendar year; the planning for this eventful year, however, began months and years before. When projecting the costs of the anticipated activities and when the involvement of national nurse and non-nurse leaders is desired, long-range planning is critical. Bringing these prominent individuals to our campus was part of meeting our goal of bringing the School of Nursing to the forefront in the university and the community.

A few of the critical issues in planning were as follows:

1. Involvement of as many different fiscal budget years as possible.
2. Utilizing regular budget allocations for specific Jubilee items—paper, program covers, coffee cups with the "logo," honoraria, etc.
3. Involvement of as many alumni members, community members, faculty, and students as possible.
4. Utilization of regular university resources whenever possible.
5. Utilization of individuals in the university with specific expertise by requesting this help of chief officers.

The keys to success of these strategies were:

1. Having all potential and desired events listed in a calendar as quickly as possible to provide a working framework and time line.

2. Identifying items like logo, theme, and specific presentations of these items *early* (sweatshirts, coffee cups, bookmarks, paperweights, etc.).

3. Identifying items to be used for one time events.

4. Identifying budget years to be used for each major event.

5. Tying School of Nursing events to regularly scheduled university events whenever possible to maximize resources (School of Nursing to lead commencement procession during Silver Jubilee year, for instance).

6. Arranging for the university Public Affairs office to emphasize the School of Nursing's Silver Jubilee during its regular scheduled events (Homecoming, Founders Day, University Honor Day, etc.).

7. Working through the regular University Speakers Series to share resources and have the university bring in a major speaker, to be designated as the School of Nursing Dean's Lecture.

8. Seeking the cooperation of the president of the university with all plans—assuring him that all plans must be tasteful, of interest to the entire community (while at the same time not overusing the theme "nursing, nursing, nursing").

9. Establishing a special revolving fund for Silver Jubilee proceeds and expenditures at the discretion of the dean.

10. Building and maintaining a data base of alumni, community leaders, university officials, politicians, and other interested parties (schools of nursing nearby) in order to keep them informed of activities and build participation.

11. Networking with other university and community leaders to utilize their speakers before and after the "main event" for which they were brought.

After all the planning and implementation of the keys to success, the following major events were scheduled for the School of Nursing's Silver Jubilee Year (all were high level and of minimal cost to the School of Nursing):

1. The annual University Founders Day is sponsored by the Alumni Affairs Office at Indiana State University. The Director of Alumni Affairs welcomed the opportunity to bring a national leader in nursing to the campus to speak with alumni, university staff, community persons, and the larger nursing community in Indiana. Dr. Pamela Maraldo was the February 1989 Founders Day speaker and will always be remembered for her excellent presentation. She was able to spend special time with students, with faculty, and with the Indiana League for Nursing members. The university alumni office paid not only for the

speaker but also for the invitations, postage, receptions, luncheon, and printed programs (with the School of Nursing Silver Jubilee logo, of course!).

2. The School of Nursing's First Annual Research Day was held in March 1988 and was sponsored by the Continuing Education Division. Dr. James Vail served as the keynote speaker for the day and the entire event was underwritten by Continuing Education participant fees.

3. The university schedules an Honor Day annually in April where academic awards are given by all the schools. For the 1988 Honor Day, Dean Billye Brown was the speaker and she was able to spend time with our students and faculty as well. The Vice President for Academic Affairs paid all expenses for this visit, since Dean Brown was the Honor Day speaker.

4. During May 1988, the School of Nursing organized a brunch for graduating students held in conjunction with our pinning ceremony. A local bank was approached and they agreed to sponsor the cost of the brunch itself for all our graduates and their families in honor of the Silver Jubilee year. We also combined the annual Alumni Banquet of our Schools of Nursing (the two local hospital schools which had closed and our Indiana State University School) as a tribute to our Silver Jubilee. The District #3 chapter of the Indiana State Nurses' Association also honors spring graduates with a banquet each year. The School of Nursing and the district organization pooled resources and brought former ANA President Eunice Cole to speak at all three of the aforementioned events. She was also able to meet with many nurses in various clinical agencies around our community.

5. In September we went all out—we organized an all-day All School Convocation involving our students, faculty, community and state leaders, and university officials. The university president underwrote the cost of flying all three former deans and their families back to Indiana State for special recognition and presented each of them with a Presidential Award at a special luncheon. Former ANA President Barbara Nichols was also brought in from the University of Wisconsin and gave an inspirational presentation to our students and faculty. That evening we hosted a gala dinner/dance at the university, complete with ice sculpture, 9-piece orchestra, black tie, silver balloons, and on and on. Patrons were solicited to help defray costs of the dinner/dance and we were able to deposit $5,000 in a special nursing student scholarship fund after the final figures were totaled.

6. Dr. Ingebourg Mauksch was the special guest for a Homecoming Continuing Education offering and costs for her trip were paid by participants in the event.

7. The University Speakers Series underwrote the very special appearance of our Dean's Distinguished Lecturer, Robert Gale, M.D. His several talks on the experience of treating victims of the Chernobyl nuclear disaster and calls for responsible public policy were standing room only.

In addition to the major events listed above, some of our other activities during the year included:

1. A book signing and reception featuring the authors of the *History of the School of Nursing* (which had been commissioned for the Silver Jubilee year and included a listing of alumni activities as well).

2. The sale of memorabilia all year long (paperweights, lapel pins, coffee mugs, sweatshirts, tee shirts, the history book, buttons, briefcases, folders)—not just to make money, but to have fun and to increase our visibility (all items included our logo).

3. The Silver Jubilee year was also designated as *The Year* to initiate the process to establish a Sigma Theta Tau Chapter on our campus. Dean Billye Brown, President-Elect of STT, met with students and faculty during her visit in April and provided the impetus needed. We have just completed the site visit phase of the process and been informed that we have been recommended to receive a charter.

4. An Opening Ceremony was held at the School of Nursing in January 1988 to kick off our year. A large cake with candles proclaimed "Happy 25th Birthday, School of Nursing!" and was cut and served by Dean Roehm and the university president to students, faculty, and staff.

5. Proclamations honoring our School of Nursing were issued by the university president, the mayor of Terre Haute, the governor of Indiana, and the Indiana legislature. Congratulatory messages were received from our national legislators as well as Dr. Otis Bowen, HHS Secretary and former Governor of Indiana.

6. Fifty large banners proclaiming the Silver Jubilee year were displayed all along Wabash Avenue in downtown Terre Haute (cost bourne by the university Public Affairs office) and several of the banks with digital sign displays congratulated the school during the September celebration.

7. Month-long displays about the history of the ISU School of Nursing were featured at the Wabash Valley Historical Museum, the university library, the Swope Art Gallery, and the local public library—all at no cost to the School of Nursing.

As we've now had a chance to look back on our Silver Jubilee year, the school is proud to have renewed our friendships of the past 25 years, to have renewed our relationship with our alumni, to have established some "firsts" that will be carried into the next century, to have honored our former deans, to have brought so many wonderful speakers and events to our town and university, and to have added money to the student scholarship fund. We were able to accomplish all these things without unpaid bills and only a few of the events involved any costs to participants at all.

Our original goals—celebrating our history, looking toward the future, increasing the visibility of the School of Nursing—all were achieved!

59

BUILDING ALUMNI RELATIONS THROUGH HISTORY

Justine J. Speer

This contribution will describe the efforts to conduct nursing history through the collaborative efforts of an academic nursing professional and professional historian.

Louisville General Hospital, the oldest diploma school in the state of Kentucky, closed in 1967. Decades before, LGH nursing administrators tried to transform the program into a collegiate school. The University of Louisville, then a private institution, admitted a class but closed it a year later because it was not cost effective. All dreams of transforming the LGH school into a collegiate school died in 1967 when another attempt failed and the school closed. If it had been successful, the nursing program probably would have become part of the University of Louisville.

As a new dean, I spent a lot of time learning about Louisville. I quickly learned the nursing stories which occurred in "old General." Many of the LGH graduates were quite elderly; some were gone. Some of the real stories were lost. I decided that we needed to have their school history written.

Too often we throw things away because they are old. Years later we wish we had them back so we could look at them and remember. Tomorrow's students need to have a historic conscience. Those women accomplished a lot with limited resources. I wanted our students to know the story of early nursing in Louisville.

I was smart enough to realize that recording history accurately is not easy and takes a lot of time. I had not been trained in the research method and I did not have the time. To accomplish the task I decided to find a professional historian who would undertake the study; I would offer my assistance if needed.

Fortunately, my first choice accepted the challenge. She was a doctorally prepared historian working for a private historical research association. We met to discuss the task and make a plan. The contract outlined the goal, our mutual responsibilities, and the cost. After I received her written proposal, I began to raise money for the project. Our direct costs would include the salaries for the historian and staff assistant, travel expenses for interviews outside Louisville, and the expense of printing our report, in total approximately $4,000.00.

To increase community support and recognize ULSON's history which started with the LGH School of Nursing, we previously had adopted 200 alumni whom we could contact. Many alumni volunteered donations for the development of the history. We submitted successful written proposals to the Kentucky Oral History Commission and the Jefferson County Medical Foundation. The University School of Nursing also donated hours of staff and secretarial time.

We assigned a staff person to coordinate all activities. This person contacted all the alumni, scheduled all interviews, and wrote letters of confirmation to all those who agreed to be part of our project. She was present at all interviews, greeted alumni, operated the equipment, obtained informed consent forms, and helped the infirm. She was familiar with historical resources available, made notes about other resources suggested, and classified memorabilia given to the school.

The historian was an expert. She knew the historical context of the years when nursing was emerging in Louisville. The staff associate spent hours searching official documents for references to the LGH hospital or its nursing school. I served as the professional expert, knowing nursing's historical issues and some of the solutions tried. Being present at most interviews, I clarified respondents' comments and facilitated discussion when necessary.

The historian was responsible for writing the final report.* I offered suggestions on content and style. The report gave Louisville General Hospital School of Nursing its place in the history of nursing. Alumni and city officials were eager to read the document.

The history gave nurses recognition for what was an important era in nursing. It also gave the ULSON a chance to build our alumni ranks and build community support for the school. In the end we all won.

---

*Jones, A. A. (1988). The Louisville General Hospital School of Nursing 1887–1967. Louisville, KY: History Associates, Inc.

Part XII

DREAMS

60

LOSE SOME, WIN SOME

Geraldene Felton

Once one becomes a dean and has entered administration as a career, one is into power and politics and dealing with other humans whose motives are endless. The dean's power is her ability to influence and persuade. To think otherwise is asking to become disillusioned and bitter.

When I accepted my first position as dean of a developing nursing program, I negotiated with central administration for three things: an administrative assistant, a budget officer, and a women's toilet on the same floor as the school of nursing's faculty offices. At this point, it is important to state that the school of nursing was housed on the first floor of the four-story Engineering Building. In the distant past, what had originally been intended as women's lavatories on each floor had long since been turned into laboratories or storage areas. The engineering secretaries (all women) were all assigned one women's lavatory on the second floor. Of course, there were men's lavatories on each floor.

When work began to convert the first floor lavatory for women (covering urinals, installing soap and paper towel dispensers, more toilet stalls, etc.), an aggressive campaign was lodged. The senior engineering faculty started to complain. The conversions were torn out. Notes were sent to the faculty union that the language of the contract was being violated. The Board of Trustees asked the university president to explain the source of the engineering faculty's complaints of harassment. The "good old boys" meant trouble.

143

Some perquisites die hard. Some never die. I had set off an emotional hot button. If you do not want to have any more problems than necessary, one has to know what is going on. Learning how to deal with problems and how to make decisions on the right amount of data are survival skills. The legitimacy and worth of conflict is how it contributes to arriving at a climate to help solve problems. I made an appointment with the president and relieved him of his promise to convert a lavatory for women. By backing down from an unacceptable goal, I not only gained support among the engineering faculty but also the reputation of being adaptable and having a sense of humor.

I learned to pick my fights carefully. At the end of 6 years, the School of Nursing had magnificent space in a beautiful new building.

It takes a lot to be a good administrator. It takes even more to survive. The dean builds bases of support—slowly—accomplishing the school's objectives and maintaining coalitions. I not only had the administrative assistant and budget officer, I had a marvelous story to tell at cocktail parties! And finally, I married one of the senior engineering faculty—a ringleader in my "problem."

61

"WALK A MILE IN MY SHOES"

Jacqueline Rose Hott

An idea that I have not yet tried is based on the indian concept, "Walk a mile in my shoes." I believe that were each faculty member to have an opportunity to do an internship with the dean for a semester—go to all meetings, on and off campus; sit in all the agonizing conferences (except tenure/promotion); help prepare the myriad reports, etc.—there would be less griping about what the dean does or does not do. I have spoken to a nurse administrator of a hospital who rotates first-line managers through her top-level administrative offices for a month each. She has found that once managers have seen "the other side," they have a better understanding of the director's problems and are more likely to deal with their own independently and to need less direction and supervision. Internships within one's own institution is something I really would like to try.

62

GENERIC NURSING EDUCATION: A GRADUATE PROGRAM

Ildaura Murillo-Rohde

My dream—something I consider a superior idea—is that I would like to see the generic nursing education program at the master's level. This is not an original idea, but ever since I worked with Dean Frances Reiter as Chairman of the Department of Mental Health–Psychiatric Nursing at the Graduate School of Nursing, New York Medical College, in such program, I was convinced that generic nursing belongs at the graduate level. I worked with Dean Reiter for 5 years in her generic master's program, and it was a great program.

The maturity and superiority of graduate students' ability to grasp concepts and deal with problems, as well as develop ideas and projects, is something nursing needs and could use in the education and formation of nurses. The master's generic nurses are better equipped to give the scientific, compassionate quality nursing care that is germane to a humanistic discipline like nursing.

Nursing is the only health profession whose programs are not always at the baccalaureate level, let alone at the graduate level. As we move into the 21st century, we need to do better. The old Yale University nursing program was a generic program at the master's level. Pace University inherited the Graduate School of Nursing's program and its generic Master in Nursing. Rozella Schlotfeldt established a generic doctoral program at Case Western Reserve University, but I feel that neither nursing, society, or even most students are ready for such program.

Perhaps the investment of time and money is too great considering what the graduates will receive in assignments and wages.

The generic master in nursing education is long overdue. Nursing, like all other health professions, belongs at the graduate level. The twenty-first century would be the perfect time for the establishment of generic nursing at the master's level. When this happens, nursing will come of age! It is my hope that I may see this before I rest.

63

THE DNSc–PHD ATTEMPT

Luther Christman

Clinical practice is applied science. Researchers, who have both a substantial insight into clinical practice as well as a very rich scientific base, have a vastly increased potential to augment the quality of clinical content needed to improve the care of patients. The combination of clinical and scientific degrees provides this base. This level of strength enhances the power of perceiving the problem in an insightful way and conducting research in a sophisticated fashion. The inherent potential for producing interesting and desirable breakthroughs is apparent. It is from this background that Noble laureates can emerge more readily.

The many and useful improvements in care that are an outcome of MD–PhD efforts are an indication of this power of knowledge. The Markel Foundation program, which existed for many years, had this goal of increasing the power of medical research as the basic premise of its funding. In Sweden, where there is a very high percentage of physicians with this preparation, the quality of care and clinical research are notable.

So far, I have only been able to interest four nurses to accept this rigorous preparation. One student had her PhD but did not have a nursing background. The other held a PhD but when he first expressed an interest in nursing, he was guided into hospital school preparation. He has finished the DNSc and is launched on what appears to be a successful research and practice career. The other candidate has not completed her clinical doctorate at this writing. Two other nurses accepted the challenge. One has finished and is with the National Science Foundation; the other is still in the throes of her effort. A number of other young nurse candidates have discussed this possibility but have not committed themselves. Unfortunately, in some cases, their faculty mentor has not been very supportive. The concept remains to be tested. No one can use knowledge he or she does not have no matter how high their aspirations may be. When I think about the strength of the research effort in the nursing profession, I wonder if only we had a hundred nurses with this form of preparation.

Perhaps someone, or some dean, will be able to influence graduate students more effectively than I could. I wish them much success.

64

LET THE COMPUTER LIMIT THE AGONIZING IN CURRICULUM DEVELOPMENT

Loretta C. Ford

Over the years, I have been struck with the time, effort, and, therefore, money that faculties and their curriculum committees waste in developing conceptual frameworks, objectives, etc. These activities are especially frustrating when one sees "the products" of these horrendous efforts. Few new, innovative, or creative ideas are generated. Sessions become psychotherapeutic persuasions (or coercions) between committee members; the costs in not only money but also frustrations and emotional trauma are phenomenal.

My idea to address this issue is for the government or professional organization to underwrite the creation of a computerized national or even international data base of philosophical components, concepts, objectives, etc., which can be tapped by any faculty member who is developing, revising, or rejuvenating curriculum.

Additionally, course sequence, the learning resources needed, faculty requirements, and costs could be projected by computer. After all, there are only so many verbs for faculty to use in the English language to describe behaviors! (Of course, we could continue to convert nouns to verbs, if necessary.)

APPENDIX A

LETTER INVITING PARTICIPATION

In the summer of 1989, Billye J. Brown will retire from the deanship of the School of Nursing, University of Texas at Austin. The Foundation Advisory Council, along with students, alumni, and faculty are planning several types of recognition to honor her for contributions she has made to our school, to the profession of nursing, and to individuals. Because Dean Brown is known nationally and internationally, through the growth of our school under her deanship and through her extensive activities and fulfillment of responsible roles in professional organizations, many nurses are interested in things associated with her. Her interests are as broad as all aspects of nursing, health care, and education. Among her interests, a major focus is administration: administration in its broadest sense, its many facets, and its continuing evolution and development.

In recognition of this interest, we shall attempt to provide an opportunity for nurses to learn about administration from the too frequently ignored past, from the working present, and from thoughts that will promote growth and innovations for the future. We shall go to the very most knowledgeable source, the deans of accredited schools of nursing in the United States. We shall ask these peers of Dean Brown to contribute to a compendium of information about the business of administration.

We are asking you to reminisce and to write a brief description of the *very best innovation you ever implemented* as dean. Please think in terms of a simple outline of the project and the results. We should like the story of

151

your best innovation, but just possibly you have had what you consider a superior idea and have never been able to implement it. The idea still has your confidence, you still think it should be tried, you think it would work. If you would rather write that description, there still be a place for it. Or you just may want to write one of each—the very best innovation and the idea that merits testing. Do it, there will be a place for both.

We perceive this project as a way for top administrators to extend their individual influences. Each will share information about one administrative success; some will describe ideas that need to be tested. The compilation of the many may be expected to encompass the broad variety of responsibilities of a dean. Such descriptions of experiences utilizing innovation in execution of some facet of administration will provide a wealth of information and inspiration for active administrators and for students.

We shall compile these gems into a book with a dedication to Dean Brown and acknowledgement of all contributors. The ideas will be organized into areas of focus, such as students, faculty, clinical facilities, university relations, alumni, budget, community relations, and others. We envision the interested audience to be deans, administrators, and students.

We hope you will view the project as worthy of your participation and as a means to convey congratulations to Dean Brown on the occasion of her retirement.

Thank you for your interest and assistance in making this a worthy recognition honoring Dean Brown.

Sincerely,

David B. McWilliams, *Chairman*

Mabel A. Wandelt, *Member*

Betty J. Thomas, *Collaborator*